Rattled

What He's Thinking When You're Pregnant

Rattled

What He's Thinking When You're Pregnant

HOGAN HILLING

TURNER

Turner Publishing Company

200 4th Avenue North • Suite 950
Nashville, Tennessee 37219

445 Park Avenue • 9th Floor
New York, NY 10022

www.turnerpublishing.com

Rattled: What He's Thinking When You're Pregnant

Cover design by Mike Penticost

Library of Congress Cataloging-in-Publication Data

Hilling, Hogan.
Rattled : what he's thinking when you're pregnant / Hogan Hilling.
     p. cm.
ISBN 978-1-59652-825-3
1. Fatherhood. 2. Fathers--Psychology. 3. Wives--Psychology. 4. Fathers and
daughters. I. Title.
HQ756.H5584 2011
155.6'462--dc22
                         2011009621

Printed in the United States of America

11 12 13 14 15 16 17—0 9 8 7 6 5 4 3 2 1

This book is also available in gift book format as
30 Things Future Moms Should Know About How New Dads Feel
(978-1-59652-760-7)

To the working wives of at-home dads for their faith, confidence, and support of their husband's role as the primary caregiver.

16. I may need you to coax me out of my "man cave" — 85

17. I'd like you to acknowledge me as your primary person of support — 91

18. It's important for you to respect my male friendships — 97

19. I'm confused about my role as a dad in today's world — 103

20. I'd like you to honor and embrace my role as the breadwinner — 109

21. I'd like you to help people respect my role as a new dad — 115

22. I'd like you to value my thoughts about the delivery room — 121

23. I don't want you to be the "perfect" pregnant mom — 127

24. I have fears about becoming a dad — 133

25. I may need your help making peace with my father — 137

26. I also have guilt trips — 141

27. I worry about the baby's and your health — 145

28. I need your help balancing time at work and home — 149

29. I need to have some reasonable "me" time — 155

30. I need help networking with other dads — 159

Introduction

For the last twenty-five years, there has been a call for new dads to be more sensitive and share their feelings about the pregnancy and their child. Most new dads have not answered the call. At the same time, new moms have continued to share their frustration about their husband's unwillingness to share his feelings. Many experts have offered their theories as to why a new dad won't wear his heart on his sleeve, from genetics to the biology of the male brain, to the way men are raised as boys to the male-female language barrier, and to men just being men. But why this is so is no longer as important as finding a way to break down this great emotional divide between new dads and moms. I wrote this book to help a new mom *get in touch* with what a new dad is feeling and bridge the communication gap.

"Every time I honestly shared how I felt about being a new dad with my wife, she showed no sympathy or turned our conversation into an argument. Eventually, I stopped telling her how I really felt."

"It's really hard to keep how you feel bottled up inside. And even harder to live with a wife who you can't turn to for support and comfort."

"I honestly shared how I felt about an important issue with my wife. But it didn't sit well with her. I was in the doghouse for a week."

Also standing in the way of a new dad sharing his feelings is the misconception he doesn't know how or doesn't have any desire to share his emotions with his wife. The truth is he does know how and wants to get what's ailing him off his chest. One of the biggest surprises I discovered in my expectant dad workshops is that most of the dads shared intimate details of how they felt with me and the other guys (who they'd just met for the first time) that they had never discussed with their wives. This was a real eye-opener and motivated me to continue my work as an advocate for fatherhood.

I'm sure you've heard the adage "Be careful what you wish for, you just might get it." Well, if you want your husband to share how he feels, then you have to be prepared to not only accept his answer but also give it the credibility it deserves and show him some sympathy. And if you really want to know how a new dad feels, then this book is for you. Here is how *Rattled* can help.

The information I provide will eliminate the guessing game a new mom usually has to play to get to the root of what is bothering her husband and any issue he may be struggling to overcome. If a new mom knows the emotions her husband is dealing with, finding the solution to whatever he is struggling with will be easier for her to work out with him. In this book, some things a new mom will learn about include how a new dad feels about being left out and isolated, his struggle to bond with the baby, resentment towards the baby, his fears about being a new dad, guilt, finances, being in the delivery room, and his mortality.

As you read this book, keep in mind that a new dad will experience some or all of the issues I listed to some degree. Some dads will accept and acknowledge them. Many dads will not. For a new dad to deny that he has any concerns or issues is not healthy. Whether he admits them or not, what is important is that you have a greater understanding of how a new dad may feel and the issues that might be of concern to him.

Once a new dad shares how he feels, don't take it literally or personally. Remember, it isn't about *how* he shares his feelings but rather *what* he is feeling. If you can stay focused on the latter, you'll make more progress in encouraging your husband to become more transparent about how he feels.

All a new dad wants is for his voice to be heard and

acknowledged. Just because he disagrees with you doesn't mean he doesn't love you. Nor does it mean that you're correct and he is wrong. A new mom and dad by the very nature of their genders view the world of parenthood differently. Neither view is right or wrong, just different. And just because a mom and dad parent differently doesn't mean they can't parent together. A good way to approach parenthood is to view parenting as two people (a mom and dad) sharing one role and not two people sharing two roles.

Also be aware that many dads will struggle with their transition into fatherhood. Some dads will figure out how to navigate through the daddy track on their own while others will struggle and feel lost. Use the information in this book to help give your husband the nurturing nudge and encouragement he needs to become the best husband and dad he can for his new family.

Before you turn the next page, I'd like you to step out of your mommy shoes, put them in the closet, and step into your husband's shoes until you finish reading the rest of the book. Although you'll never know what it's really like to be a dad, I believe this book will help you accept how it feels to be one.

1
I still want to be your main squeeze

Do you remember the day you fell in love with your husband? Most women do. You also probably remember what he and you were wearing. It was a special day for both of you, and the beginning of your life together as a couple. Then he proposed to you. You said yes.

Do you remember why your husband married you?

Do you remember why you married your husband?

I think it was so that each of you could be the number one person in the other's life, for better or worse, until death do you part—not till baby do you part. As husband and wife, you were his main squeeze and he was your main squeeze. No other woman could have him. And no other man could have you. Your marriage is and should be the most important thing in the world. Without the commitment to place each other first before any other person, there is no marriage.

Then one day your life changes again for the better. You and your husband decide to have a baby. Becoming a mother and father and starting a family was one of the many dreams you strived to create and have shared with each other. Now that you're pregnant, the dream is about to come true. You're going to have a baby. Or are you?

You're probably thinking, *What a silly question! Of course I'm going to have a baby.*

Yes . . . and no.

Yes, you're pregnant, but with an unborn fetus. The fetus is not technically defined as a baby until after the birth. Now you may feel I'm being petty. But bear with me. There is a valid point I'm trying to make that will benefit you and your husband in the long run.

For all purposes, the unborn fetus has been referred to as the "baby" since the beginning of time. I'm not trying to take away the joy that comes with a woman being pregnant and becoming a mom and a man a dad, but the reality is that both of you are delivering another human being into this wonderful world. Therefore, you are not just inviting a baby into your life but also a third person.

Whatever love you gave to your husband must now be shared with a third person—the baby. This is not an easy thing for a man to accept. I know many fathers who have experienced feelings of resentment during and after the pregnancy. A man may perceive the baby as a threat to his relationship with his wife. As a result, he may distance himself from both you and the unborn baby by making excuses to not attend the doctor's appointments, help with the household chores, or attend the baby shower. You may perceive his actions to mean he is not feeling excited about being a dad, when in fact, he feels a lack of love from you. And he doesn't want to tell you how he really feels because he doesn't want to hurt your feelings and upset you during the pregnancy. He fears that any emotional turmoil could hurt the baby. This is an example of how men sometimes demonstrate compassion by not saying or doing anything, and of how the way a new dad acts sometimes gets lost in translation. (I'll elaborate on this in Chapter 16).

As far as a husband is concerned, he was in his wife's life before the baby. A wife needs to give this fact the weight it deserves. He was his wife's first main squeeze, and he doesn't want to lose that title. If you place the baby before your husband, it is normal for a man to feel some level of resentment towards the baby.

Don't get me wrong—a mother should express love for a baby, but not at the expense of her husband's love. If your love for him doesn't have the same intensity it had before the arrival of the unborn baby, he is not going to give that same love to you or the unborn baby in return. If not, his resentment could damage the marriage and his experience of fatherhood.

To help you relate to what your husband might be feeling, imagine how you might react if he placed his mom ahead of you and then justified his actions by saying, "I'm sorry you feel that way, but I have only one mother. She gave me life, so I should put her needs before yours."

Or how would you feel if your husband chose to attend an NFL football game with his friends over accompanying you to a social event like a play or concert or a doctor's appointment. I'm certain you would be a little upset and feel as though you aren't as important to him as you thought.

I'm not suggesting that a wife always consider placing her husband's needs first at all costs. There will be special circumstances when you will need to choose another person's needs before your husband's. What's important is that you and your husband have an understanding that he is and will always be your main squeeze. What is also important is that your relationship as husband and wife doesn't change during and after the pregnancy.

Now that you're pregnant, there really are three different relationships going on. Husband and wife. Mom and baby. Dad and baby. Maintaining three relationships is quite a juggling act that will require the stability of a strong husband-wife relationship to foster the growth of a new family.

Be careful that you don't get so preoccupied with being a new mom that you neglect your husband. If you let the baby bleed your relationship with your husband, it may cause him to feel useless and disconnected and could eventually strain your marriage.

A new mom can also get so caught up in the hype of the pregnancy that she forgets how important her husband is to her and to the baby. In case you get sidetracked, here is a list of reminders to keep you on track.

- Your husband is the one who helped you create the baby. You wouldn't be a mom without him.
- If your husband is the primary breadwinner, he is the one paying the bills, not the baby.
- If your husband will be the at-home parent, you will count on him to care for the baby while you're at work. Therefore, he will be the most important person in your life, not the baby.
- If you and your husband both work, regardless of who earns more, his income along with yours helps pay for the bills. Not the baby's.
- Your husband will be your primary person of support, not the baby.
- Your husband is the one you will need to count on after the birth, not the baby.
- If your husband is the handyman around the house, he will be the one you turn to for repairs, not the baby.

The baby is dependent on both of you. When a mom is not available, the next person in line is dad. If you place the baby before your husband, you may push him to resent the baby, resulting in him giving less of himself to both of you.

If you're still skeptical about the importance of placing your husband before the baby, consider the rising divorce rate and the reasons marriages fail. Some of the main reasons husbands separate or divorce include neglect and lack of intimacy from their wives. If you don't want your new family to become another divorce statistic, do your part to insure that your husband is and always will be your main squeeze. After all, don't you want him to do the same for you?

Yes, your husband is now a dad. Nevertheless, he is still your husband first. Forge a strong bond with your husband and focus on your relationship with him. Do whatever you can to strengthen your bond with him. As you strengthen the bond with your husband, so, too, are you helping him strengthen the bond with the baby.

Being a mom should not get in the way of your relationship with your husband. The spotlight should be on your marriage first and then the baby.

Be a wife first, then a mom. As one dad noted, "I wish my wife would talk to and treat me like I'm her husband first and then our baby's dad."

2
I may not act as excited as you about the pregnancy

While a new mom is often accepting of the pregnancy as soon as it is confirmed, acceptance is a major emotional and developmental task for a new dad throughout the pregnancy. His first step is to accept the reality of the baby, which can be difficult since the baby is something he cannot see, feel, or touch. As the pregnancy continues and more concrete evidence of the baby becomes available, such as hearing the heartbeat or seeing the ultrasound, the father begins to gradually accept the pregnancy. With each passing day, his new identity as a dad begins to hit home, and his transition into fatherhood, unlike that of a new mom's into motherhood, progresses at a snail's pace.

When you shared news of the pregnancy with your husband, there was a brief moment of shared excitement. Did

After I received news of Tina's pregnancy, I was thrilled about it, but my joy was short-lived. The reality of becoming a new dad was surreal and overwhelming. I wasn't into the ceremony of the pregnancy and cuteness and tender moments Tina was thinking about in a life with our new baby. I became apprehensive and started questioning whether I was prepared for fatherhood. One concern after another popped into my head. I walked around like a zombie trying to sort out the details of my future life as a new dad. Like most dads, the first two things I worried about were the finances (I'll address this topic in more detail in Chapter 13) and all the things that could go wrong with the pregnancy and birth. While I was preoccupied with these two issues, other concerns popped into my head that included lifestyle change, my wife and baby's health, bonding, how to choose a doctor, sex, managing the household, balancing work and family, isolation, my mother-in-law, handling advice, sleep deprivation, and day care. It seemed like a never-ending list. One day I would have four of these issues on my mind and then the next day, four, five, six, or seven different ones. I spent more time worrying than enjoying the prospect of being a new dad. I believe I represented how most men feel after hearing news of the pregnancy.

Here are comments that dads made about some of the concerns I listed.

"My wife says she can't wait to meet our baby. Me, I'm worried about the lifestyle change I'll have to make."

"I'm worried about my wife having a miscarriage. She's been dreaming of this moment since our engagement three years ago. I don't want her to be disappointed."

"I recently started a job with a new law firm. Expectations are high, and I'm worried about how I'm going to balance work and time with my new family."

"While my wife is wrapped up in the joys of the pregnancy, I'm worried about how I'm going to pay the medical bills and balance my life at work and home."

If your husband gives you the slightest impression that he isn't as excited as you or dreads becoming a dad, don't take it personally. What he is feeling is as normal as the joy you feel in becoming a mom. It's just going to take a little time for him to catch up to you. Be patient and do what you can to help him feel the joy of being a new dad.

3
I know you're pregnant, but the baby also belongs to me

Pregnancy is a biological condition that nature bestowed the honor of to the female gender. A woman is the one with the uterus, vagina, and other body parts that enable her to become pregnant. It is one of the greatest privileges of being a woman. A man is not allowed this honor. Women get pregnant. Men don't. That is the nature of life.

But despite the prestigious honor of carrying and growing a baby in her body, pregnancy can do crazy things to new moms that baffle new dads to no end. One battle most men struggle with is the possessive behavior over the unborn baby their wives develop during the pregnancy. Whether it is intentional or unintentional, most new moms convey a message to the new dads that the very nature of the pregnancy gives them full ownership of the baby. The attitude is that it's my body and I should have the final say in what is best for the baby.

Possessive behavior is a silent killer that can plague a marriage. It manifests itself in a variety of ways. Some of the ways include a slip of the tongue when the new mom refers to the growing fetus as "my baby" in conversations; takes full control of the decisions related to the pregnancy like which doctor, hospital, childbirth class, or birth method to choose; controls who can and can't be involved during the pregnancy and dictates this to her husband and other family members; or makes a dad feel inept in front of relatives, doctors, childbirth instructors, friends, neighbors, and strangers.

Possessive behavior can also cause emotional harm. It can cloud a new mom's ability to have empathy for her husband. And that is not fair, because if a new mom expects and desires empathy from a man, she must give it in return. Lack of empathy can also lead a husband to resent or feel disconnected from the unborn child, make him feel excluded, and most important, discourage him from being an involved dad.

There is an old adage that states, "Possession is nine-tenths of the law." Whatever you possess is yours until someone legally proves otherwise. In the case of an unborn baby, our society has determined that the fetus belongs to the mother because she is in possession of the baby. But a new mom does not have to buy into this legal perspective. What she needs to buy into is a dad's perspective. It may seem trite to make this distinction, but don't you want to do everything you can to make your husband feel more connected to the baby and become the best dad he can be? Here is what some dads had to say about this topic:

"I told my wife how her behavior was making me resent her as a mom. I wished she had never gotten pregnant. Not because I didn't want to be a dad, but how the pregnancy brought out the 'dark side' in her."

"In my wife's mind, the baby belonged to her because she was carrying it. She had to be in control of every aspect of the pregnancy. The more I tried to get involved, the more she pushed me away. And the more I felt disconnected from the baby. It was as if I could only be involved in the pregnancy on her terms. If she is this possessive about the baby now, what will it be like after the baby is born?"

"I don't think my wife realized how possessive she was about our unborn baby. When I mentioned it to her, she flipped out. I never shared how I felt again. I ho-hummed my way through the rest of the pregnancy. After the baby was born, my wife became even more possessive. It took months for her to leave the baby alone with me."

"My wife's possessive behavior and baby mama drama is making me feel that I'm being robbed of fatherhood."

To plead my case for the new dads, pretend for a moment that you hired another woman to be a surrogate mom. All parties involved—surrogate mother, you, and your husband—agree in a legal contract that after the birth, the surrogate mom will give up the baby, and that you and your husband will become the legal parents and retain ownership of the baby. During the pregnancy and according to law, the baby belongs to the surrogate mother because she is physically carrying the baby in her (not your) uterus. Like your husband, all you have is an emotional investment in the baby. Your role is to support and assist the surrogate mom in every aspect of the pregnancy, just as your husband would do if you were pregnant. At the end of the nine months, you expect to be rewarded with possession and ownership of the baby. Despite nine months of developing an intense bond with the unborn baby, the surrogate mom shows great character, integrity, and strength by relinquishing ownership of the baby to you and your husband as per the contract agreement. The point I'm making here is that if a woman can relinquish her bond with a baby for another woman, she is also capable of doing the same for her husband.

Of course, there is the possibility that some surrogate moms will be reluctant to hand over the baby to the intended mom and dad as agreed upon in a legal contract. It's a legal nightmare that no parent would like to experience, but it happens. This scenario, however, is no different than a biological mom not honoring her contract to equally share ownership of the baby with her husband and biological dad of the baby.

The pregnancy is supposed to be a joyous occasion for a new mom and dad. However, it can quickly turn into an emotional nightmare for a new dad when a new mom makes her husband feel as though he has no ownership of the un-born baby. But when a new mom relinquishes equal owner-ship of the baby to a new dad, it will inspire and empower him to be more involved. And isn't that what you want for yourself and the baby?

The reality is that after the birth, the baby will be shared not only with the dad but also with relatives, neighbors, and friends. Feel free to cherish and relish the honor bestowed upon you to carry the baby, but always remember that the baby also belongs to your husband.

4

Your miscarriage is also my miscarriage

The first three months are a scary time for new moms. Since over 25 percent of pregnancies will end in a miscarriage during the first trimester, a new mom has reason to worry. New moms count the days and pray the baby lives until the second trimester, when the chance of a miscarriage drops dramatically. Nevertheless, the thought of a miscarriage is still of concern throughout the pregnancy. And not just for the new mom.

Although a new dad's anxieties can't compare with those of a new mom, the thought of a miscarriage is just as devastating and painful for a new dad. When it does occur, the immediate response of others is to express compassion and sympathy for the new mom and dad, but just as it is with the news of the pregnancy, it isn't long before the spotlight turns to the new mom, and the new dad is yanked off the stage and forgotten. Relatives, friends, and neighbors naturally focus their attention on the mom to comfort her and provide her with emotional support. After all, she is the one who was carrying the baby and had to deal with the unpleasant side effects of the miscarriage that include vaginal bleeding and passing of blood clots, which further complicates the feeling of loss for a new mom. Soon after the miscarriage, a mom can become so caught up in her grief that she unintentionally forgets that her husband is also grieving.

I attribute this behavioral trend to the nature of our culture. Unfortunately, there is a tendency in our society to not show the same level of sympathy and empathy to new dads as to new moms, as if to suggest that a mom's bereavement is more painful than a dad's, and that a new dad's bond to the unborn baby that he has worked so hard to establish had no value. In our culture, a man's role in the death of a loved one is to be the rock and the person giving emotional support, not receiving it. Well, guess what? The loss of life is equally as painful for a man as it is for a woman. A man also needs a shoulder to lean on, as these dads came to realize.

"A few days after we received news of the miscarriage, I was still pretty distraught. I wanted to talk to my wife about it. But after I saw how much more distraught she was, I decided to just be there for her and worry about me later."

"I received the usual sympathetic words. But as the days passed my wife was receiving all the attention. She was also receiving cards expressing sympathy for her loss. I was left alone to lick my wounds."

"We already had names for the baby. The dreams I had hoped for as a dad suddenly vanished. It made the loss much more difficult."

"The miscarriage happened so fast. I was a proud dad-to-be. Then all of a sudden our baby is dead, and I'm not a dad anymore. Next thing I know, my job is to console my wife. But nobody is around to console me."

"I worked hard to bond with our baby. And now she is gone. Yet, people act as though I had no invested interest or relationship with the baby. I'm also grieving, but my wife has received most of the sympathy and hugs."

"It has been six months since the miscarriage, and I'm still grieving the loss of our baby and being a dad."

I think the reason there is a tendency for people to show more sympathy towards a new mom is that the mom is pregnant, and they view the miscarriage as synonymous with pregnancy loss. I don't have a dispute with the fact that mom is pregnant. I am arguing that what has really occurred is the loss of a baby, especially if the baby already had a name. And also lost are dreams. Lost dreams of motherhood and fatherhood, watching a child grow and play sports, graduate high school and college, maybe get married and have children, and especially for some dads, a broken dream of adding a branch to the family tree.

Now there are circumstances in which a new dad may not experience the same level of grief, with reasonable explanation. The bond between a baby and mom is unique because the baby is growing inside her womb. This bond begins the moment a new mom receives news of the pregnancy, whereas a dad may not begin to develop a bond with the baby until seeing the ultrasound picture or after the baby is born. This means your husband may be less affected by the loss. This doesn't mean his loss is any less painful but rather that his grieving period is shorter than a new mom's. So don't get upset at your husband for not showing the same depth of grief. It may be taking him longer to come to terms with the loss of the baby.

As I noted in Chapter 2, mom is pregnant, but the baby also belongs to dad. The same is true with a miscarriage. Just because a dad doesn't experience the symptoms of a pregnancy or a miscarriage doesn't mean he is immune to the pain and grief. The gain that once was is now a loss for both mom and dad.

If you and your husband are one of the 25 percent who experience a miscarriage, my sympathy goes out to both of you. As you mourn the loss of the unborn baby, please don't buy into the myth that men don't acknowledge the death because they are afraid of the hurt and aren't emotionally equipped to mourn the loss, or that men will not accept help and support. Men are equipped to grieve. People just don't give new dads the compassion and sympathy they deserve. Give your husband a little more credit because he is also grieving. And if both of you are still struggling with the miscarriage, please read other books that address this issue or seek counseling.

For the 75 percent of the new moms lucky enough to not experience a miscarriage, I encourage you to turn the page and continue reading about how a new dad really feels about the pregnancy.

5
Pregnancy nation is all Greek to me

A new dad knows very little about the biology of a pregnant woman and even less about pregnancy. Pregnancy is as alien to him as football can be to a new mom. While first-time moms have some basic knowledge of pregnancy by the very nature of their gender, most new dads are at a disadvantage when it comes to pregnancy. To most new dads, pregnancy territory is a foreign country. In order to acclimate to pregnancy, a new dad must learn more about the culture, geography, and language.

The culture of pregnancy can be quite a shock to a new dad because he will be asked to do things outside his comfort zone. Although culture shock can be perplexing and scary, it is a normal process every new dad goes through. For some it happens all at once, and for others it is a gradual process.

As a new dad, he will need to learn how to deal with what I call the "cultural baggage" of pregnancy. Cultural baggage includes the customs of pregnancy and the values that are important to a new mom and dad as well as the patterns of behavior that are customary in their family's tradition. The customs of pregnancy may include carrying a pillow from the car, through the parking lot, and into the hospital lobby, elevator, and childbirth classroom; shopping at the Babies R Us store; or following the correct protocol when people ask questions about the pregnancy. It is normal for a new dad to experience some level of discomfort before he can function with a degree of confidence in his new setting and not develop a complex about carrying a pillow in public. With regards to the values of a family, a family's tradition in the U.S. will be different than those of families in Italy, Japan, Mexico, Thailand, India, or Germany. If a new dad is in an interracial marriage, it can create some unique challenges that may also make it uncomfortable to acclimate to the pregnancy.

When it comes to the geography of pregnancy, a new mom has an internal GPS system that gives her a sense of direction to find her way through the pregnancy landscape. A new dad doesn't have any kind of guidance system available to him. He is left to fend for himself and navigate through the female-dominated world of pregnancy on his own. And even when he finds his way to the doctor's office, hospital, family resource center, and childbirth classroom, he must deal with another obstacle—the language barrier.

Learning another language, for most people, is extremely difficult and takes great commitment. In the world of pregnancy, all the road map information is written in a new mom's native tongue: Venusian. And there is no Venusian to Martian dictionary or interpreter available to help a dad decipher pregnancy's complicated language. The ABCs of pregnancy are filled with unfamiliar jargon and medical terms that often make a new dad feel uncomfortable about the pregnancy. Like a traveler in a foreign country, even after learning the basics of the language, it takes time for a new dad to acclimate to his new environment.

Unlike what a new mom receives, there is no welcoming party or mentorship program to help a new dad feel at ease. Nor is there an information center to give him the direction and guidance he needs to help him become familiar with the lay of the land. A new mom also has the advantage of turning to female friends for help and advice. A new dad generally doesn't have male friends he can rely on for assistance or guidance in this area.

I believe almost every new dad wants to learn more about the pregnancy and will be a good learner. All he needs is a helping hand from a trustworthy person to point him in the right direction, teach him the vocabulary, and make him feel comfortable about the pregnancy. And the right person for the job is the new mom.

Although a new mom may already feel overwhelmed having to carry the baby, it is in her best interest to help a first-time dad become more familiar with his new surroundings because what he doesn't know about the pregnancy will hurt him and eventually the baby. The best thing a new mom can do is to get a new dad to a point where talking about the pregnancy comes naturally to him. The sooner he establishes a comfort zone, the better. If a new mom can help a new dad learn to love the pregnancy, the pregnancy will love him back. If both of you can accomplish this feat together, think how much love both of you will receive after the birth of the baby.

6
I may struggle to bond with our unborn baby

Bonding is the bedrock of a person's emotional develop-
ment and an important element in building a relationship with another human being. Building a relationship is
a process that occurs between friends, girlfriend and boy-
friend, and husband and wife. Some of these relationships
last a lifetime. Some don't and eventually lead to breakups,
friends parting ways, or divorce. The mom-and-baby bond,
however, seems to have a much greater longevity because of
the genetic tie and nine months of sharing the same body.

There is an assumption and a high expectation in our
culture that mom will develop an immediate and blissful
bond with the unborn baby and that a new dad is expected
to follow suit. Both assumptions are far from the truth and
unfair because there is more to bonding than meets the eye.

There are many new moms as well as dads who struggle to bond with the unborn baby. There are many reasons for this, including carrying unresolved emotional baggage, feeling overwhelmed by the responsibility, or simply not wanting to be a parent. The latter occurs more often in an unplanned pregnancy. Needless to say, the pressure placed on mom and dad to establish an immediate bond with an unborn baby is intense and unreasonable.

A new mom can get so caught up in her desire to bond with the unborn baby that she forgets how complex it is. Bonding with a baby is a personal experience that takes time. For a new dad, it is not a "love-at-first-sight" experience. There is also no one-size-fits-all magical "Super Glue" bonding formula. Another truth is that there are many first-time moms who feel indifferent or ambivalent about being pregnant. These moms may develop feelings of shame or inadequacy. There are also new moms who don't bond at all. This is confirmed by moms who put the baby up for adoption and the many stories that have been printed about a mom abandoning her newborn baby in a dumpster. Despite the unfortunate tragedy, people tend to be very forgiving towards the mom.

New dads, however, don't receive much of a break. They are at a disadvantage because they don't have the physical connection moms have to the unborn baby. It isn't fair that a new mom and other people make such a big deal when a new dad doesn't build a bond with the same intensity or enthusiasm or at the same time as a new mom does. There is also the perception that if a new dad doesn't bond immediately that something is wrong with him, when in fact, his behavior is quite normal.

"My wife threw a fit just because she didn't think I was bonding enough with the baby."

"I was just as frustrated as my wife that I couldn't bond with the baby. But I didn't need her to tell me that something was wrong with me and that I need to see a psychiatrist."

"I wish I wouldn't have told my wife that I was having trouble bonding. Now she is upset and thinks I don't want the baby."

After the news of the pregnancy, there is a lot that goes through a new dad's mind that triggers aftershocks. These aftershocks come in the form of anxieties like:

- *Resentment:* This is not the type of resentment I noted in Chapter 1 about a dad being jealous of the unborn baby, but rather that of a dad questioning his choice to become a new dad. He may experience periods of feeling inadequate about becoming a new dad. How much this affects him will be based on the relationship with his father (which I will cover in Chapters 25 and 26).

- *Finances:* A new dad may start to worry about how he will pay the medical bills. Some may even start to have anxieties about paying for college tuition. Especially in a down economy, a bleak future exacerbates his anxiety. (I will cover finances in more detail in Chapter 13.)

- *Lifestyle change:* Marriage is quite a commitment, and husbands and wives have periods in which they fall in and out of love with each other. This is also true with a baby. A new dad may love the baby one minute for the joy it will bring into his life, and the next minute resent it for the financial burden and effect it will have on his marriage.

- *Mom and baby's health:* If a new mom and baby experience some unexpected health issues, it may delay a new dad's ability to bond with the baby. The struggle to bond becomes more of an issue if the doctor determines that the baby will be born with a disability or deformity.

In addition to these anxieties, a new dad has a major obstacle to overcome that a new mom doesn't have to address. A new mom has a direct connection to the unborn baby via the umbilical cord. Since she is the unborn baby's lifeblood, she has a vested interest in developing an emotional connection with the baby. A new dad, however, is unable to build a relationship with a nontangible object that he can't see or touch; his brain is not wired to function on a spiritual level or without some kind of tangible, positively reinforced behavior or reward. What a new dad can't see he can't feel. What he can't feel he can't measure or find gratification in. A new dad will even struggle to bond with the baby after the birth for the same reason, because newborns don't do much but eat, sleep, and poop. There again, a new dad, and even a new mom, will experience some level of delay in the bonding process with the baby. A new dad, unlike a new mom, will need to train himself to find ways to spiritually connect with an unborn baby. Therefore, the bonding process will take time.

For some parents bonding is immediate. And if it is for you, consider yourself lucky. But for most new moms and dads, it takes a little more time.

If your husband is one of the latter, be patient. The more pressure you apply, the more resistant he may become to bond with the baby. Instead of forcing him to bond, address the reasons he isn't first and then find ways to help him make a stronger connection with the baby. Also, remember that if you don't work on bonding as husband and wife and strengthen that relationship first like I noted in Chapter 1, it will be more difficult for a new dad to bond with the baby. The new dad and baby bond will be only as strong as the bond that exists between a husband and wife.

7
I need more time than you to adjust to the pregnancy

Pregnancy for a new mom is the real deal for obvious reasons. For a husband, the reality of officially becoming a new dad doesn't register in quite the same way. His reality check doesn't set in to his brain until after the birth of the baby. This hampers his ability to adjust to the pregnancy as quickly as a new mom.

I feel a common mistake new moms make is they forget pregnancy is a dramatic first-time experience for new dads as well as for themselves. This oversight can result in new moms also overlooking the enormity of the adjustments new dads need to make during the long, stressful, nine-month pregnancy. The oversight can also spark a new mom to place some of the same unrealistic expectations on a new dad as she did around his bonding with the baby.

Do you remember your "first times"? First car. First job. First marriage. After the euphoria of doing something for the first time fades, the anxieties of how this new venture will affect your life kick into gear. As each day passes, you have to make adjustments and take on more responsibilities in the life you've chosen with your new car, job, or spouse, like paying for car insurance, gas, maintenance, health insurance, food, clothing, and housing. The same is true when it comes to pregnancy and parenthood.

Pregnancy is a major culture shock for a new dad. The adjustment from singlehood to husbandhood pales in comparison to the transition into fatherhood. Instead of juggling life and relationships with two people, he must now do it with three people. With the adjustments come many anxieties, because each decision he makes involves consequences that will reshape his life as a new dad. A new dad wants to be the best husband, dad, son, son-in-law, employee, student (in the childbirth class), and friend during the pregnancy. But dads can't be all things to all people. Neither can moms, which I will cover in Chapter 23.

A new dad's life is already hectic before the pregnancy. Now he has to squeeze in more responsibilities and duties in the same amount of time. A new dad stumbles through the pregnancy just like a new mom. Oftentimes he is blindsided with an array of adjustments, and unlike a new mom, when he trips up, everybody notices and points it out. He feels like he is always under the microscope, which places even more pressure on him to adjust to the pregnancy. Making adjustments takes time and is not going to happen at the snap of a finger. Adjustments also have a domino effect. If a dad makes an adjustment in the workplace, it will affect his personal or social life and vice versa.

Here is an example of the domino effect. A new dad agrees to the new mom's request to spend more time helping with the household chores, which means less time at the office. Now that he is spending less time at work, his job performance suffers. His employer brings it to his attention. Further complicating matters is his friendship with one of his buddies who invited him for a round of golf. A new dad is suddenly faced with a no-win dilemma. If he doesn't spend more time with the new mom, he'll be in the doghouse. If he doesn't perform better at work, he may lose his job and his income to provide for his new family. If he says no to the golf date, he may lose a close friend. There is a solution to this problem, but it will take time for a new dad to work it out. (See Chapter 28 for the solution to the employer problem, and Chapter 18 for the golf solution.)

A new dad needs time to weigh the pros and cons. And just when a new dad feels comfortable and satisfied with the adjustment, another adjustment must be made. The adjustments are never-ending, and the baby hasn't even been born yet.

One major reason it takes a dad longer to adjust is that people are much more willing to make compromises and attend to a new mom's needs than to a dad's. Two examples are

the difference in social attitude towards maternity and paternity leave and the support services available for new dads
compared to moms. (Other examples are noted throughout
the book.)

Although some companies offer paternity leave, many
men do not take advantage for two reasons: one, because
political pressure was the true driving force behind providing the leave rather than a sincere intention to support new
dads, and two, because behind closed doors the message to
a new dad is that his job will be in jeopardy if he elects to
request paternity leave. How is a new dad going to provide
finances for his family to pay the bills if he has no income
during his leave of absence?

The second example involves support services for dad,
which are minuscule compared to those available for new
moms. A new mom has access to abundant resources and
information, including a multitude of books, Web sites,
childbirth centers, and family resource centers, and she
also has access to people who serve as guides and mentors
to tell her what she should know about and do during the
pregnancy. These people include her mom and other female
relatives, female friends, family doctor, OB-GYN, childbirth
instructors, and doulas. When new mom requests help, almost everyone comes running at her beck and call, only a
phone call or e-mail away, offering assistance. Sometimes a
mom receives help even before she requests it. That is how
readily available support services are for new moms.

However, even if a new dad does reach out to request

help, one of the following occurs. Those who hear his request, almost always female, have no knowledge or information on how and where to find help for a new dad. Or the new dad is not offered any assistance because none is available. Or the new dad's needs are ignored. Or the new dad is told to man up.

Despite the lack of support, most new dads march on and do their best to adjust to the pregnancy. Just think how much easier it would be for a new dad if he received the same level of sympathy, resources, and support that's available to a new mom.

8
I'd like you to respect my title as Dad

Comedian Rodney Dangerfield developed a catchphrase that launched his career and earned him the admiration of his peers and audiences. Dangerfield's monologues began with "I get no respect." Ironically, Dangerfield received respect by joking that he never got any respect. He made himself the butt of his own jokes and laughed all the way to the bank.

Most new dads also feel they get no respect. Unlike Dangerfield, new dads don't laugh all the way to the bank. Instead, they suffer emotional bankruptcy from all the unfair ridicule they receive about their performance on the daddy stage. To new dads, fatherhood is no joking matter. Yet they continue to be the butt of jokes when it comes to parenthood. They want to take their role seriously, but how can they if people, especially new moms, don't take them seriously and continue to perceive them as bumbling idiots?

Why is it that people don't respect fatherhood in the same manner as motherhood? How did this lack of respect for fatherhood develop? I believe the answer lies in people's misinterpretation of the word "respect," and the unfortunate myth about men as dads.

I feel most people today miss the boat about the true meaning of respect. Somehow the standards and value of showing respect have been lowered and turned into a lost art. I believe the true meaning of respect is showing that you value the office or position of another person, and at times either courteously yielding to the person's perspective or at least showing empathy. For example, a person may not respect the man who is the president but still respects the office of the presidency. Regardless of his or her political affiliation, that person still addresses the man in office as "Mr. President."

People, in general, hear what they want to hear and see what they want to see, based on their beliefs. If you're a new mom and have been given the impression since childhood that men are bumbling idiots when it comes to fatherhood, then you will probably believe it, and eventually, the only way you will perceive a new dad is as a blundering, uncaring, inept dad. In desperation, a new mom resorts to making futile attempts to fix him, which only results in making him more inept. Men don't need to be fixed. What they need are words of encouragement and mutual respect.

I feel fatherhood doesn't receive the same respect as motherhood because more credit is given to her as the one who carries and gives birth to the baby. This fact of nature should not devalue fatherhood, but it has. To devalue fatherhood this way is no different than a new dad overstating the significance of his role as the primary breadwinner. The status of both mom and dad is equally important but in different ways, and both deserve mutual respect. Unfortunately, fatherhood still lives in the shadow of motherhood. And there is ample evidence to support this claim.

Our culture and the media have not been kind to fatherhood. In 1984, Hollywood's release of the movie *Mr. Mom* stigmatized men as inept primary caregivers. The *Mr. Mom* tag stuck and sparked a wave of movies that portrayed fathers as absent, incompetent, or dangerous, like *Three Men and a Baby* and *Daddy Day Care*. Subsequently, dads have become the target of jokes that make them look increasingly foolish.

Then in 1996, fatherhood took another devastating hit with the release of the book *Fatherless America: Confronting Our Most Urgent Social Problem* by David Blankenhorn. Blankenhorn's book brought public attention to the notion that fatherlessness was the leading cause for America's social ills.

Fatherlessness is the most harmful demographic trend of this generation. It is the leading cause of declining child well-being in our society. It is also the engine driving our most urgent social problems, from crime to adolescent pregnancy to child sexual abuse to domestic violence against women. Yet, despite its scale and social consequences, fatherlessness is a problem that is frequently ignored or denied. Especially within our elite discourse, it remains largely a problem with no name.

If Blankenhorn had written this paragraph about motherlessness, I wonder how people would have responded to its message.

There is such a negative image in our culture of men as fathers that it is easy to see how a new mom can be skeptical about a new dad's ability and performance and show little respect for him.

Are we to believe that fatherlessness in families is caused only by a father's decision to leave his family? Are we also to believe that mothers never play a part or aren't guilty of contributing to or even initiating a divorce? Should we believe that moms are not capable of abandoning their children? I don't think so.

As I noted in Chapter 6, there have been many stories about moms who have abandoned their babies in dumpsters. There are also moms who have murdered their children. Two unfortunate incidents are the mom who drove her car into the lake with the children buckled into their car seats, and the mom who drowned her children in the bathtub. Moms are also just as capable as fathers when it comes to committing adultery, having a drug or alcohol addiction that leads to destroying a family, and creating social ills. But I have yet to find a book that addresses the negative impact a mother's absence has on society. Nor have I found any literature that bashes or criticizes motherhood in the same vengeful way it has fatherhood. Despite the continued father-bashing, there is one refreshing movement that has dispelled the Mr. Mom myth. And that is the increasing population of at-home dads.

Just as women have proven that they can be productive wage earners in corporate America, so, too, have at home-dads shown men can be competent primary caregivers for their children. According to statistics, the number of at-home dads in the U.S. varies. There is no true number because many at-home dads are afraid to come out of the pantry, struggling to accept and publicly announce their role as the primary caregiver for reasons I will explain in the next chapter. The size of the population, however, is not as important as the positive impact the at-home-dad family trend has had in communities across America. Not only have the children benefited, but so have the moms; this new family lifestyle has allowed them to pursue their careers and become the primary breadwinners. At-home dads even have their own organization, Daddyshome, Inc., complete with a resource and support system. The organization also hosts an annual At-Home Dad's Convention. More information about Daddyshome, Inc. can be found at www.daddyshome. org.

Al Watts, Vice President of Daddyshome, Inc., stated on www.momaha.com, "I believe that dads should share the parenting pedestal with moms and be treated as equal parents. They should be valued and respected for their parenting role rather than ignored and ridiculed."

There is a saying in sports that there is no letter "I" in the word team. A husband and wife is a team. A new dad and a new mom is a team. One of the philosophies I instilled in players when I coached youth basketball is that when you respect and help your teammates become better, you also become better as an individual player and as a team. History has shown that even great players cannot win championships without the respect and support of other players. The same is true with marriage and parenthood.

What a new dad would like from his wife is for her to respect his title of Dad.

9
I don't want to lose my masculinity

Mother Nature did a terrific job designing a woman. I love everything feminine about my wife, Tina, especially the pregnancy part. There is no way I'd want to experience what it feels like to carry and deliver a baby. I'm happy to be a man. I was attracted to Tina because she was feminine. And Tina was attracted to me because of my masculinity. At no time in our marriage have I asked Tina to show her masculine side, nor has Tina asked me to show my feminine side. To do so would be to take away part of each other's identity and dignity as man and woman, husband and wife, mom and dad.

One of the biggest blunders made in our culture has been suggesting that men show their feminine side. Mother Nature created a man and a woman differently for good reason. Besides, it isn't nice to fool Mother Nature. Unfortunately, many people have been fooled into believing that a man has and should show his feminine side—not based on fact but rather based on a supposition pulled out of thin air. The truth is that men don't have a feminine side. Nor do women have a masculine side. Another truth is that I have yet to hear of a campaign that asks women to show their masculine side. I'll also bet that most men have no desire to have relations with a woman who has a masculine side.

Today, many men are very confused about their male identity and even more about being a dad. They have been fooled and pressured into believing that to be a good man, husband, and dad, they have to show a feminine side that is totally unnatural for them. But this request comes at a huge cost for a man because it means he has to lose part of his masculinity. In essence, a man doesn't feel like a whole man. When a man doesn't feel like a whole man, his spirit and self-esteem are damaged. Eventually, he loses his desire to be the best man, husband, and dad that he can be.

Despite the good intentions of this campaign to feminize men, it has emasculated and harmed fatherhood. It is not possible for a man to be masculine if he is acting like a woman. To suggest that the only way a man can be successful as a nurturer and caregiver is to show his feminine side is insulting to both a man and a woman. There is a huge difference between asking a man to show his feminine side and asking him to be caring and sensitive. Who determined that emotions like caring and sensitivity were synonymous only with females? The truth is that they are not. Men have feelings, as this book demonstrates. And men can be just as compassionate, sensitive, and caring as a woman and still be a hundred percent masculine. Let's use the role reversal in corporate America and the at-home dad lifestyle as an example.

When corporate America's good ole boys club finally accepted women into the workforce, they gained recognition for their accomplishments and were rewarded handsomely with promotions and substantial salary increases. Many of these women ended up in high-level management positions. Are we to believe that these women's accomplishments were attributed only to their masculine side? To do so would not only discredit these women but also send a message to other women that the only way they can reach the same accomplishment would be for them to show their masculine side. I feel the same way about my role reversal as an at-home dad.

When my wife and I chose the at-home-dad lifestyle in 1991, people were quick to criticize us. Tina was criticized for allowing a man, her husband, to be the primary caregiver and choosing career over children. Many people also felt that a female nanny or a day care—not the father— was the optimum alternative. I was criticized for not fulfilling my role as the primary breadwinner and choosing my kids over a business career. That I volunteered (I wasn't getting paid) to be the primary caregiver demonstrated my ability to be compassionate, sensitive, caring, and thought-ful, traits that people considered feminine. But they are not. These traits also exist in men but in a masculine way.

People also assumed that I was incapable of being a nurturing, loving, and competent primary caregiver and wouldn't last long. When I did prove that I was capable, people credited it to my feminine side. I nurtured, cared for, and managed the household like a man, not the way my wife would have. I changed diapers like a man, sometimes put-ting them on backwards. I dressed my kids like a man and didn't color-coordinate them. I multitasked like a man, and by the end of the day, the house was in good order. Every aspect of my at-home-dad life was done with a hundred per-cent of my masculinity. There was nothing feminine about me. I still drank beer, smoked cigars, watched sports, and played poker.

I didn't choose to be the at-home parent to be a replace-ment for a mom. My twenty years as an at-home dad proves that you can take a man out of his masculine role but you can't take the masculinity out of a man. Likewise with wom-en, as evidenced by the increasing population of women in Fortune 500 management positions. A woman may be in what people consider a man's role, but she still puts her panty hose on one leg at a time.

I hope you can see how this "men-showing-their-femi-nine-side" campaign has spun out of control, and that noth-ing good has nor will come from it.

Masculinity is important to a man just as femininity is

to a woman. Let's not devalue either gender. This gender difference is also important to a baby because after the birth, he or she will need a mom and a dad—not two moms. Most men want to be a macho man and want their kids to see them as a macho dad. So please stop looking for a new dad's feminine side. It's a mythical beast that doesn't exist. Don't try to inject your husband with a feminine side. Don't destroy the core of his being. Don't let him stray from the intrinsic qualities you admire in a man. And don't fear your husband's masculinity. Instead embrace, respect, and nurture it. And when you do, it will increase his chances of blossoming into an awesome dad.

10
I'd like you to acknowledge me as an equal partner

In my book *Pacifi(her): What She's Thinking When She's Pregnant,* I noted that the biggest challenge a man faces as a new dad is his EGO (Everyone's Greatest Obstacle). A new mom also has a similar obstacle she may not be aware of: hogging the spotlight of the pregnancy.

No doubt about it: pregnancy is a special, beautiful, wondrous endeavor reserved for a woman. But when a new mom steals the spotlight and takes full credit and control of the pregnancy, it makes a dad feel his role during the pregnancy is not equally as important as hers. Often, a new mom believes her role is more important just because she is the one experiencing the medical complications of the pregnancy and carrying and being kicked by the baby. This is an unfair position to take because a new dad is equally as valuable as a new mom.

If a new mom expects a new dad to share an equal interest and investment in the responsibilities of a pregnancy, then she must acknowledge and treat him like an equal partner. An equal partnership cannot be accomplished if one person feels that he or she is more important than the other. This is why it is so important for a new mom to respect the title of Dad (see Chapter 8). Without the respect, a new mom cannot treat a new dad as an equal partner. What I mean by equal partners has nothing to do with keeping track of the amount of work or tasks each person performs. This is not about keeping score but rather about acknowledging the contributions a person—in this case, a new dad—brings to the success of a partnership.

A new dad shouldn't be penalized just because he can't carry the baby. What a new dad brings to the parenting table may be different, but that doesn't mean it's less valuable. For example, in a traditional marriage (whether single-income or two-income), the breadwinner provides the money to pay the bills for a new mom's maternity clothes, doctor visits, and childbirth classes. Another example is division of household chores. New moms tend to discredit or downplay the manly chores around the house. If you have a husband who is also an excellent handyman, then chores like mowing the lawn, repairing a faucet, taking out the garbage, building a room addition, or assembling furniture are just as important as washing dishes, mopping floors, and vacuuming the carpet. If you have a husband who is not, then be grateful if his earned income can pay for a gardener, handyman, or maid.

When it comes to household chores, most new moms stir up controversy with unrealistic expectations and focus too much on how and not what duties a new dad performs. I'll bet in most households that after a new dad completes a task, a new mom is quick to criticize how the job was not done the way she would have done it. Unfortunately, the human urge to criticize another person is much stronger than the tendency to acknowledge or praise a person. This is especially true between husbands and wives. And when they become new moms and dads, it becomes even more prevalent.

What a dad should receive is a compliment and more time to hone his skills. And speaking of compliments, most new moms flatter their girlfriends more than they flatter their husbands. A new mom needs to ask herself which is more important: Husband or girlfriend? *How* a new dad cleans the house or that he actually did? That a new dad offered or even did something should be worth at least a few kind words of praise.

Most new dads feel that they don't receive enough acknowledgments from a new mom for all the little things they do, and that much of her time and energy is directed towards what he isn't doing right. Imagine for a moment what it would be like if a person followed you all day and only pointed out all the mistakes you made and didn't acknowledge any of your accomplishments. A perfect example of this type of person is Ray Barone's mother, Marie, in the show *Everybody Loves Raymond*. Marie prides herself on being an exceptional mother, cook, and housekeeper. She never sees herself as being overbearing or critical of other family members. And she dismisses anyone who doesn't live up to her standards, especially her daughter-in-law, Debra. Marie often criticizes Debra for not keeping her house clean and orderly and not feeding her family properly. Marie is a constant emotional thorn in Debra's side. Most new dads feel the same way about new moms because they are quick to criticize and slow to praise.

Just like new moms need to be acknowledged, so, too, do new dads. Praise will go a long way to motivate a new dad to do more and improve his skills. And the more a new mom acknowledges a new dad, the less likely she will be to turn into a Marie Barone.

11

I will also have mood swings and a bumpy ride

One minute a new mom is on cloud nine because of the pregnancy. Then without warning she behaves uncontrollably like a screaming banshee. A new dad is taught to accept and tolerate her tirade, understand she may not have control over her emotions, and dismiss it as being caused by the pregnancy or PMS.

One minute a new dad is caught up in the joys of fatherhood. Then out of the blue, something sets him off to the point of frustration. When a new mom is the target of a new dad's tirade, she views it as inappropriate behavior or emotional abuse. Instead of showing sympathy and attempting to understand the cause of his frustration, she offers advice on how he needs to take control of his emotions, seek counseling, or attend an anger management class. Imagine how you would feel if you received the same response and advice from your husband. I don't think you'd take too kindly to his opinion.

Well, guess what? A new dad can also be under the influence of PMS—Pregnancy Mood Swings. New dads also have mood swings. But when a new dad loses his cool, we chalk it up to a bad day at the office. However, researchers have concluded that men may also suffer from a chemical imbalance in their bodies identified as Irritable Male Syndrome (IMS). According to American psychotherapist Jed Diamond, IMS is as real and damaging as any of the hormonal fluctuations that affect women. Diamond has written a book, *The Irritable Male Syndrome,* based on his own experiences and those of the thousands of men who have written to him or visited his California clinic. He defines IMS as "a state of hypersensitivity, anxiety, frustration, and anger" that occurs in males. Sound familiar?

A new dad's mood swings can be unpredictable and vary in intensity. He can experience a wide range of feelings, from joy about the pregnancy and the prospect of finally holding the baby, to anxieties over finances and ambivalence towards fatherhood. Emotions and reactions likely to surface can include frustration (often mistaken for anger), fear, stress, insecurity, impatience, and fatigue. A new dad can also experience symptoms like headaches, weight gain, insomnia, and nausea, all common anxieties and symptoms of everyday life that are exacerbated by the pregnancy.

Although there is no evidence to prove chemical changes

in a new dad's body can cause moodiness, there are other factors that can make a new dad feel down in the dumps. In addition to financial concerns and ambivalence towards fatherhood, other anxieties can also include pressure and stress from work, unrealistic demands by new mom, lack of intimacy and sex with wife, an overbearing mother-in-law, concerns about mom and baby's health, adjustment to a new lifestyle, lack of attention from childbirth instructor to address his concerns and needs or a comment that questions his manhood or ability to be a good dad, or unresolved issues of life with his father and/or mother.

A new dad may be unaware of the change in his mood or triggers of his grumpiness. He just feels the urge to blurt out his frustrations. Due to the nature of the beast, he is a walking time bomb with suppressed feelings that can explode at any minute. When a new dad does release his frustrations, a new mom can misinterpret his emotional tirade as uncontrollable anger and rage. Generally speaking, almost every man's bark is worse than his bite. All new dads want from new moms is the same courtesy a new mom expects from her husband when she goes topsy-turvy and verbally lashes out at him—an open ear, acknowledgment of their frustrations, a little sympathy, and a hug. (Please note, however, that if a new dad's frustration manifests into uncontrollable anger or physical abuse, it is time to seek counseling.)

Life before pregnancy was quite an emotional roller coaster ride. Now with the impending birth, the ride will get even wilder with unpredictable mood swings that will test the resilience of a new mom and dad. There is no way to avoid the bumpy ride, but a new mom and dad can do their best to stay on track and make the most out of what the ride has to offer. The greatest challenge will be how a new mom and dad deal with the emotional ups and downs. Remember that both of you will be wrung out by the demands of the pregnancy, so you need to find the strength to be there for each other.

One day a new dad may be riding high while a new mom may be at a low point. The next day a new mom may be on the high end and a new dad, the low. In each case, the person at the top needs to act as the safety mechanism that helps keep the other on track. And when you experience the high moments together, make sure each of you takes the time to cherish them, because it will be these moments that will give both of you the strength to continue on this emotionally charged pregnancy journey together.

12
I'm not a mind reader for females

If you really believe that a man is capable of reading a woman's mind, I have a bridge and swampland to sell you. A man does not have the psychic power to read a woman's mind or any person's mind for that matter. Nor does he have any desire to know everything that is on a woman's mind because some thoughts are better left unsaid. However, if he were lucky enough to have extrasensory perception bestowed upon him, he wouldn't waste it on a woman. Instead, he'd use the telepathic power for monetary gain and head to the nearest casino.

What a new dad also doesn't want from his wife is to play the game of hint-a-husband charades. History has shown that new dads don't play this game very well. They have a tough time matching answers with their wives on *The Newlywed Game.*

For the sake of argument, let's pretend that a new dad can read his wife's mind. Let's also keep in mind she is pregnant and suffering from bouts of PMS. How can he possibly satisfy a wife who is experiencing mood swings and constantly changing her mind every nanosecond? How will it be possible for him to know what a new mom is thinking when she doesn't even know when her next unpredictable PMS outburst will occur? If a new mom has little or no control of her emotions, how is a husband supposed to decipher the message and make sense of what's going on in her head when she doesn't even know? Confused? So are new dads.

Scientifically speaking, a man can't read a woman's mind and vice versa because their brains are wired differently. They also function differently. One of the differences is that a woman's brain operates on emotion and a man's on logic. Furthermore, there is no scientific proof that a human is capable of psychic powers, although some people have tried to deceive us into thinking they are clairvoyant. (These professionals—we call them illusionists, mentalists, magicians, or con artists—lead you to believe that they can live inside of your head for a brief moment when they really can't.)

Now I do buy into the notion that a woman *sometimes* knows what another woman is thinking and also that a man *sometimes* knows what another man is thinking. Like minds think alike. However, it is too much to ask of a man to think like a woman or a woman like a man, just as I pointed out in Chapter 9 about asking a man to show his feminine side.

So then how did this whole notion that a man should be able to read a woman's mind or know what is expected of him develop? Sometime, somewhere, somehow the communication barrier broke down. As a result what we have here is "failure to communicate."

Here are two scenarios that demonstrate how a new mom's Morse-coded message is lost in translation.

Scenario #1

A pregnant mom, Debra, is in her third trimester. The baby is due in three weeks on February 12. It's Super Bowl Week. The new dad, Cameron, asks his wife whether it's okay for him to attend a Super Bowl Sunday party at his friend's house. Debra says yes. Cameron is thrilled and tells his friend he'll be there. For the next few days, Debra goes into passive-aggressive-behavior mode and tries every hint in the book to convey how upset she is at Cameron for his plans to attend the party. Unfortunately, Cameron doesn't get the hint because he is so excited about the party. After he returns home, Debra wastes no time dumping her rage on Cameron: "You are such a jerk! Why did you go to the party? I'm the one carrying the baby and you're not even here to comfort me. Instead you'd rather be with your friends. I thought you loved me. Don't you really want to be a dad? What's going to happen after the baby is born?"

Scenario #2

After a long day at work, Jennifer, in her second trimester, begins cleaning the house. When Russ arrives home from his job, he grabs a beer, sits down, and watches television. Ten minutes later, Jennifer places a basket of clothes fresh out of the dryer near Russ. Another ten minutes later Russ is still watching television and the clothes haven't been folded yet. An irate Jennifer, who had a rough day at work, stands between Russ and the television with her arms folded and says, "How long are you going to sit there and watch television? Do you think the clothes are going to fold themselves? Can't you see that I'm cleaning the house and I could use a little help? What is the matter with you?"

In both cases, the new dads have been the victims of "mama drama" and led to believe that they are the problem, when, in fact, they honestly don't even understand what they did wrong. As a result, Cameron and Russ feel they are being nagged for no reason.

In the first scenario, Cameron had asked Debra whether he could attend the Super Bowl party, and she said yes. After further discussion, Debra finally admitted that she was angry with Cameron just for asking the question. She felt Cameron should have known better than to ask. But that isn't a fair argument because Debra could have said no. Almost every dad I know would have honored his wife's answer. And if the dad doesn't, then the new mom has a good reason to be upset.

In Russ's case, Jennifer had forgotten about an agreement she had made with him. Russ reminded Jennifer that she agreed to let him have thirty minutes of downtime when he arrived home from work. As for Debra's desire for Russ to help her, all she had to do was ask, "Russ, can you please fold the clothes while you're watching television? I'd really appreciate your help." And she could have also followed it with a kiss.

Telling Cameron no and giving Russ specific instructions would have taken less time and energy, and more important, would have avoided a major marital conflict. That time and energy is also better served nurturing the marriage.

In both cases, it was unrealistic for Debra and Jennifer to expect their husbands to be mind readers. The new moms also failed to communicate what they really wanted from their husbands. Most new dads want to help their wives. Just ask or give your husband *specific* directions. Don't be vague. Give it a try. I think you'll be pleasantly surprised. You have nothing to lose and will increase your chances of gaining a better husband and new dad.

13
Our financial situation is a huge issue for me

The traditional image of a dad as just the primary bread-winner has given way to an expanded role that involves a more hands-on approach in every aspect of the pregnancy. Today's dad is much more interested and invested in responsibilities beyond being the wage earner. A new dad doesn't just pay the medical bill; he also attends the doctor's visit with his pregnant wife. He doesn't just arrive home and plant himself in the recliner or on the couch; he also helps with the household chores. He doesn't just pay the hospital bill; he is also in the delivery room. But this newfound, refreshing image of fatherhood hasn't changed the way a new dad feels about his sense of duty or the anxieties that come with being the financial provider. A new dad will still make whatever sacrifice he can to fulfill this obligation, even if it means missing time with his new family. A new dad's identity as the breadwinner is very important to him, and a pregnant wife should never downplay or take his role as a financial provider for granted, even if her husband is an at-home dad or she earns more money than he does.

Regardless of the family dynamics, every day, from the minute a new dad wakes up to the time he falls asleep, his mind is filled with anxieties about his family's finances. Sometimes he even dreams about it. What does he worry about? He worries about his job security. He worries about feeding his family. He worries about how the extra expenses will hinder his ability to pay the mortgage or rent. He worries about whether he will be able to pay the medical and hospital bills. He worries about the credit card debt. Some dads will even begin to worry about paying for college tuition, prom, and a wedding. The laundry list of concerns goes on and on. He cannot escape the financial anxieties. Every day he worries about some financial matter that may affect the quality of life for his new family.

Even with health insurance, pregnancy can be a very expensive journey. According to the U.S. Census Bureau, an expectant couple can expect to pay an average hospital bill of $5,000 to $10,000 for the birth of a healthy baby. If medical complications arise, the expenses can increase to as high as $200,000. Then there is the anxiety of the added expenses after the birth. The fixed costs can include diapers, formula, clothes, day care, and other miscellaneous items. As the baby grows, so does the budget. All the little things start to add up to big dollars. Eventually, the pregnancy exacerbates a new dad's concerns about finances and may lead him to view his bundle of joy as a bundle of debt, which, as I noted in Chapter 2, may result in him not being as excited about the pregnancy as you are.

> *"How do I keep up with the bills that are mounting on my fixed income?"*

> *"I'm already working overtime to earn more money to pay off our current debt. Meanwhile, my wife keeps handing me more bills to pay."*

> *"My biggest issue isn't my fixed income but rather my wife's uncontrollable spending habits. She feels like she deserves the best of everything. Each time I look at the credit card bill, we get further in debt."*

> *"Because of the slow economy, I had to take a cut in pay to keep my job. While I feel lucky enough to still have my job, my new family and I have to live on less."*

As I'm writing this book, America is in a huge debt crisis. Economic growth is slow, the unemployment rate is high, the foreclosure rate is high, and consumer confidence is low. I'm not trying to scare anyone—I'm just stating the facts. Therefore, by the time you read this book, financial concerns may have increased dramatically for many new dads. Most expectant couples, even those who planned the pregnancy, were probably already saddled with debt beforehand. Life as a husband and wife was tough enough; now it will be even tougher with a baby in the oven.

While the future may look bleak, there is no need to panic. New expectant couples will find ways to survive. So what can a new mom do to alleviate some of a new dad's financial anxieties? I say "some" because it is impossible for most couples to achieve financial freedom. Here is a list of basic creeds you can follow that will help relieve some of your husband's financial anxieties.

- A new dad takes great pride in his earning power. Therefore, don't downplay his role as the breadwinner or take it for granted.
- A new dad's earning power is limited. Therefore, it's not about how much he earns but what a couple spends. There is a budget for every level of income. All the little things you can cut from your expense sheet will add up to less money you'll have to subtract from your husband's income.
- A new dad can't control his wife's spending. Maintain a strict budget immediately. Don't procrastinate. Take inventory control and write every financial detail on paper. You need to know what you've got, what you need, and what you don't need. Exercise self-control—don't overindulge in purchasing, and resist advertisements that solicit you with incentives to buy products

you really don't need. When you purchase an item on sale, it is still an expense.

- A new dad doesn't have access to financial aid like moms do. A new mom often has direct contact with people who either offer to help or can help relieve some of the financial stress. One example is the baby shower. If people ask what you would like as a gift, suggest they pool money with other people for the following big-ticket items or services: crib, changing table, rocking chair, or dresser; or maid service, gardener, prepared food delivery, or diaper service.

If you are at a crossroads and don't have the knowledge to come up with a budget plan, it may be in your best interest to speak with a financial adviser. If you can't afford one, there are many nonprofit agencies that have this service available.

Most new dads are good, hardworking husbands who want nothing but the best for their families. Every new dad, including me, would like to provide a kingdom without financial woes for his pregnant wife. But the reality is that it isn't possible for every new dad to fulfill this dream. Therefore, the best thing you can do is to deflate some of the pressure he feels in his role as the primary breadwinner. So take a step back and measure your husband's heart. If he is a good man, then all the material things don't matter.

14
I'd like the medical staff to be father-friendly

New moms have told me they wish their husbands would show more interest and enthusiasm about attending doctor's visits and childbirth classes. They also noted how frustrated they were with their husbands' attitudes and conduct.

> "I was so frustrated with the way my husband behaved at the doctor's office. He acted as though he wanted to be somewhere else and didn't say much or ask any questions."

> "After our second visit, my husband felt it was a waste of time for him to take off work and attend the doctor's appointment with me."

"I had to force my husband to attend the childbirth class. Once we arrived, he pouted the whole time and couldn't wait for the class to be over."

"What's the point of having my husband accompany me if he is not into the childbirth classes as much as I am?"

There is a reasonable explanation for a new dad's behavior and indifference towards doctor visits and childbirth classes. And it has nothing to do with his lack of desire. Most new dads are happy to accompany their pregnant wives and want to learn more about how to be a better husband and dad.

The problem isn't your husband but rather the way medical professionals greet and treat new dads. Like I noted in Chapter 8, the health-care experts have also been indoctrinated with the false perception that new dads are uncaring and inept. They, as well as moms, also assume that a new dad is uninterested and ignorant about the pregnancy and impending birth based on his body language. The truth is that what you see is a new dad feeling uncomfortable about his new environment. Remember "first times" from Chapter 7? When a person attempts something for the first time, there is a period of uneasiness. Once a person develops a comfort level, they quickly adjust and adapt to their new environment. In a new dad's case, however, his discomfort is compounded by the fact that the health-care industry is not father-friendly. There is well-documented evidence to prove this claim, one of which is an admission by the health-care industry of their need to implement better practices for father inclusion and their request for guidelines on how.

As I noted in the introduction, I'd like you to take a moment and step into your husband's shoes as you read through a list of what a new dad sees when he enters the doctor's office, hospital, and childbirth class. But first let me explain why medical professionals don't treat new dads with the same respect and courtesy they do new moms. All medical professionals spend years of educational training to pursue a career in health-care, during which time they are taught to service the needs of a new mom and baby, also known as the patients. They have been so conditioned to treat mom and baby as patients that they have forgotten that dad is also a patient. Not only is he a patient, he is also a customer paying all or part of the medical bill. This huge oversight by the medical professionals not to create a father-friendly environment is inexcusable. In essence, they are being disrespectful to the new dad.

Now let's take a brief look at the pregnancy landscape. I think it is fair to say that 80 to 90 percent of the professionals in health-care education and social services are women. For a new dad to enter an industry or room dominated by women is just as intimidating for him as it was for the women who first walked into corporate America's good ole boys club. When the personnel running the show don't show a new dad any respect, make him feel as though he is invisible, and don't attend to his needs, he is probably not going to have any great desire to return, and if he does, he will not be enthusiastic about it. Instead, he will begrudgingly cooperate to please his expectant wife.

Here are a couple examples of unfriendliness the medical industry can show to new dads.

When a new mom walks into the waiting room, she receives red carpet treatment. A new dad, however, is treated like an escort at the Academy Awards as he promenades alongside her. The OB-GYN staff members are usually women. And they've had no formal training on how to greet new dads. As he sits down, there is nothing in the room to connect him to his role as a new dad. No pictures on the walls of a dad. No magazines for dads to read. Yes, there are parenting magazines, but again that industry is also focused on servicing moms. Then when he sits down with the doctor in the exam room, the doctor makes no eye contact with him, and all the questions are directed to the new mom. In some offices there isn't even a chair for dad to sit in, so he is left to stand or has to ask for a chair.

At the hospital a new dad is greeted by female-dominated staff who hand out orientation literature loaded with information for new moms. In the childbirth classes, most of the curriculum is mommy-baby based. Classes for new moms and baby outnumber those for new dads by as much as ten to one. This ratio exists only in hospitals that do provide an expectant dads class, which only meets once a quarter or once a month; at the numerous hospitals without this kind of class, the ratio is even worse. After a new dad arrives at a childbirth class, he is often referred to as coach, partner, cheerleader, or significant other in the name of political correctness. All this does is make the title of Dad appear insignificant. I, and many other dads, find this offensive because we represent the majority who committed to creating a family as part of a marriage and deserve to be referred to as "dad" and "dad" only, because that is who we are.

I've also heard new moms and childbirth instructors complain that new dads don't talk or share their feelings in class. The fact that childbirth instructors file this complaint proves that they have not received formal training on how to interact with new dads. New dads don't speak up for legitimate reasons. Here are a few.

1. They don't want to upset their pregnant wives.
2. Most new dads are very uncomfortable sharing intimate information with a group full of pregnant strangers and their husbands.
3. What the childbirth instructor or new moms think might be relevant information may not be important for new dads.
4. A new dad might also struggle to find the right words to express what's on his mind, and by the time he chooses to voice his opinion, the childbirth instructor has moved on to another mom-related topic.
5. New dads don't feel a connection to a female instructor. After all, what would she know about being a dad?

Father-friendly should be synonymous with customer-friendly. When you and your husband dine at a restaurant, do you not expect both of you to be greeted and treated with equal respect? If the host and waiter acted inappropriately towards you or the cook didn't prepare the entrées you ordered to your satisfaction, would you return to that restaurant? Wouldn't you want your husband to go to bat for you? If "yes," "no," and "yes" are your answers, then I hope you will do your part to encourage the health-care industry to make changes in the way they treat and service new dads.

Medical professionals play an important role in determining how actively involved a new dad will be during the pregnancy because they will spend an enormous amount of time with your husband. Therefore, addressing this issue immediately is crucial to the future of your new family. The only way to change how people treat a new dad is for his wife to go to bat for him and advocate changes for a father-friendly environment in the home, health-care industry, and workplace. Given the same circumstances, I think your husband would do the same for you.

15

I will need some sexual healing

For single men, sex is a steamy topic, and most of their conversations about it turn into a bragging or joking session. Rarely does a single man talk about sex as seriously as he should.

For new dads, however, sex is a very serious topic. I didn't realize how serious until I started facilitating open-discussion groups with new dads. Another surprise was that I didn't initiate the conversations about sex—the dads did. As attendance and demand for the workshops grew, so did the dads' interest in discussing the issue of sex in more detail. What caught my attention wasn't the increased demand to talk about sex but rather how the dads were discussing it with each other. Every dad who spoke up was deeply in love with his wife. Their frustration wasn't lack of sex, per se. Believe it or not, it was lack of intimacy from their wives.

In a man's world, sex and intimacy are synonymous. So are the words in a court of law when the following question is proposed to a female witness: "Were you ever intimate with the defendant?" I don't know how or when women distinguished the two as being different. Webster defines the word intimate as "marked by close acquaintance, association, or familiarity," but also as "of or involved in a sexual relationship." A woman can't get any closer to having intimacy with a man than by having sex with him.

I'll bet that in most marriages, there were periods in which the sexual activity decreased before the pregnancy. And the only reason for the increased sexual activity in recent months was because of the pregnancy. So what you have isn't a lack of sex issue but a communication problem. Before I address the communication issue, I want to briefly address the science of sex, because doing so will give you a clearer picture of how and why a man feels the way he does about sex. I truly believe that understanding the differences will bring you and your husband closer. (As you continue reading, keep Chapter 1, "I still want to be your main squeeze," in mind.)

Most women have a difficult time understanding how powerful a man's sex drive is and also why he can't control it. The sex drive is there for a reason—to procreate. Since a woman only ovulates once a month, a man has to be ready at a moment's notice to fertilize the egg. To help a man be on twenty-four-hour call, nature designed him to be more sexually driven than a woman. In 2005, one of Britain's top sex experts told the media that in general, men are on a "five-day cycle" where sex is concerned, whereas women are more likely to be on a "ten-day cycle."

Emotionally, however, the truth is that a man thinks about and would like it more often—even more than his body would allow. The other truth that isn't discussed is that a man has no control over his sex drive in the same way a woman is at the mercy of PMS. I'll illustrate my point with a conversation I had with my wife, Tina.

"Sometimes I'm not in the mood to have sex for two reasons. One is because of PMS. The other is because my body is overstimulated, and the last thing I want when you come home is to be touched."

"I never considered touching and fondling you during the pregnancy would affect you that way."

As Tina pointed to her breasts, she said, "It's also not easy walking around with these things all day."

After Tina shared her two cents, I shared mine.

"While you have to deal with PMS, I'm struggling with MSB."

"What the heck is MSB?"

"Multiple Sperm Backup. Sometimes my scrotum is packed with too many sperm. And some of them need exercise. Sex is also a way to work off the stress in my life. Plus it's fun."

"I never viewed sex as a stress reliever. I enjoy sex but not as much as you do, so sometimes it becomes more of a chore rather than a pleasurable experience."

As I pointed to my groin, I explained, "Try walking around with this thing between your legs. My life isn't easy with *it* around. *It* has a mind of its own. I have no control over *it*. Sometimes *it* has two to three erections a day. I get so frustrated dealing with it there are days when I wish I could unscrew it and hang him up on the wall for a time-out."

Tina and I accepted each other's explanations and points of view.

What I also learned from our open and honest conversation was that I also needed to exercise some self-control and accept the idea of abstinence for a short time. There is a good chance your husband will also come to the same conclusion, but not unless you open the lines of communication. Since our conversation, Tina and I have had a healthier sex life than most married couples.

Another frustration a new dad has is how a wife uses sex as an extortion racket to force him to do more housework. I don't recommend that you use this strategy because it will turn into an inescapable tug-of-war. A dad will reply with, "Well, if you have more sex with me, I'll do more housework." In the end, neither of you win.

In the bigger scheme of things, a new dad isn't asking for a lot—just a few minutes to make whoopee. Even if you're not in the mood, give him a quickie and do your best Meg Ryan impersonation from the movie *When Harry Met*

Sally—fake an orgasm. Before you know it, he will be satisfied and so will you.

In no way do I suggest that a pregnant mom submit to her husband every time he requests to do the hanky-panky. There is a time to say "no." What I hope you will learn from the conversation Tina and I had is the importance of communicating with your husband about sex. As much as your husband may say he would like it seven times a week, it is unrealistic for him to make that kind of a demand, just as it is for you to suggest he become abstinent for the next eight months. Communication will help you find a compromise together. Talking to each other openly and honestly about sex will be cheaper than counseling sessions with a therapist.

Remember, sex is what brought you together. And sex is what will also keep you together.

16

I may need you to coax me out of my "man cave"

In the 1960s there was a common cartoon trailer that depicted a Stone Age man hitting a cavewoman over the head with a primitive club, then dragging her by the hair into a cave. This mythical animated sketch of a caveman's mating behavior (a.k.a. wife capturing) bears no resemblance to prehistoric history or to today's courting ritual because in today's "man cave," a woman is not allowed.

In 1992 a reporter coined the phrase "man cave" while writing a story about a man's remodeled basement. The man designed and built his modern grotto as a shrine of temporary refuge from his wife. The man cave was a place with some degree of seclusion he could call his own where he could spend time alone or in the company of like-minded men and have the freedom to do what he wanted to do and not worry about putting the toilet seat down. The man cave also has a set of rules to keep it manly. Since publication of the article, men have expanded places they call their own to include an office, garage, gym, golf or tennis club, a bar, lodge, room, or church.

While many wives complain about a husband's request to call a place his own or become a member of an existing man cave group, his interest to join an elite club of men is no different than a woman joining a women's support group at a family resource center, hospital, park, or church. Women need a place of solitude where they can be alone or hang out with like-minded women. Unfortunately, sexual politics has led many women to become paranoid by dubbing a man cave as a "woman-haters club." Honestly, if your husband hated women, why did he marry you? Why did he decide to help you become a new mom? Why does he return home to you after he visits his man cave? Because he loves you!

A man cave is not just a sanctuary for a new dad to hang out with his single buddies to drink beer, watch sporting events and TV shows, play poker, and smoke cigars. The man cave also serves as a think tank. Even if a new mom does not allow her husband to have or visit another man cave, he can create a fictional one inside his head. If your husband is walking around the house looking confused or dazed, it's because he has programmed his brain to make space for his imaginary man cave. Since there is no real support system available comparable to that available for new moms, a new dad may have no choice but to seek refuge inside his head.

So why does a man retreat into a man cave, and what does he do in it? It is common for a dad to have fears but uncommon for him to openly talk about it because of the "macho" factor. While some new dads are able to express their disappointments and frustrations, others don't wear their heart on their sleeve; they store it in a cave, not necessarily to avoid or hide it, but to revisit it some other time and try to find a resolution.

A new dad's retreat into his mental sanctuary can be triggered by insensitive remarks or lack of attention that make him feel inept, unwelcome, or ignored by people like his employer, coworker, OB-GYN, childbirth instructor, relative, friend, and yes, even a new mom. Examples noted in previous chapters were a new mom's mood swings, new mom's lack of desire for sex, childbirth instructor's use of the word "coach," OB-GYN's ignorance of the need to address and acknowledge a new dad, or pressure from his employer. Inhibitions and reservations about becoming new dad can also prompt him to withdraw into his man cave.

Inside the man cave, a new dad uses the time to escape the stress of life as a new dad, forget about his problems for a brief moment, heal an emotional wound, or weigh the pluses and minuses of an issue and then try to resolve it. And if he can't resolve it, he'll revisit the problem another time.

Thinking like a woman, you may feel the urge to do one of three things when your husband retreats to his man cave. The first is simply to acknowledge something is wrong, which is okay. The second is to pressure him to share what is on his mind and talk about it with you. This is not good for several reasons. Most new dads don't like to talk things out. They like to contemplate and hopefully figure it out for themselves. He may also feel there is no sense in telling you what is on his mind because he feels it is a dad issue you can't relate to or understand, so why even bring it up? It may also be that he has shared a dad issue with you before, and your response didn't warrant bringing it up to you again. If a new dad says nothing is wrong, it doesn't mean nothing is wrong. It means that he doesn't want to discuss it with you.

Whatever reason he gives for not talking about something, you shouldn't take it personally. He is wired differently than you. While it is natural for women to talk about things, some men like to ponder for a while before talking. In my open-discussion groups with dads, it may take some dads an hour before they feel comfortable saying something in front of the group. Some don't even talk throughout the whole session but still express their gratitude for having the workshop available to them. Neither I nor another dad in the group may have helped solve one of his issues at that time, but there is a chance something he heard in the group will solve a problem for him sometime in the near future. I know this to be true because I've met dads who, after attending my workshop, have said, "Hogan, that tip I got from the group—I get it now. And it's working. Thanks." So if your husband isn't willing to share and remains silent, don't take it personally. It may not be an issue about you. At some point, however, he will need to open up and discuss his concerns with you.

The third thing you may think about doing is to follow your husband into his man cave. This is a big no-no. You don't want to go in there anyway. Something inside his cave may offend you, or he may say something that you will misinterpret and get your feelings hurt. Think of it this way. You never take honey out of a bee's nest while the bees are in there. You will get stung. Instead, you coerce the bees to vacate the hive with smoke and then take the honey out.

Which brings me to what a new mom should do if her husband goes into his man cave. Coax him out like you would the bees, but don't use smoke. Coax him out with his favorite food or drink or six-pack of beer, or with tickets to an event he enjoys, like a football game, car show, theater, or hobby trade show. You can also do something as simple as mailing him a thank-you card at his place of work or buying him a personalized "Dad" T-shirt or gift. With the thank-you card, be sure to write specifically what you're thanking him for. If you feel up to some hanky-panky, wear some sexy lingerie. Help him feel like a man again so he'll know that he is loved.

An alternative to getting him out is to assure him that you value his perspective. All you need to say is something like, "Honey, I realize I haven't been very open in accepting your opinions and perspective. I apologize for the way I've reacted. Your feelings and opinions do matter. If you'll share how you really feel, I promise that I will listen and value your opinion."

A third alternative is to send a male friend into his man cave. Ask one of his friends to invite him out somewhere. Or hook him up with one of the new dads you've met at the childbirth class. (I'll discuss the importance of this suggestion in Chapters 18 and 30.)

If you still struggle to accept your husband's man cave, remember many women also have their personal sanctuary—it's called a journal.

If none of these suggestions work, that's also okay. Do something for yourself and stay busy. He'll come out soon enough. Besides, you can't keep him from entering his man cave because sometimes he does need his alone time. But you can minimize the amount of time he spends in it.

17

I'd like you to acknowledge me as your primary person of support

With all the hoopla of the pregnancy and emphasis on building a birth support team, one important matter most new expectant parents overlook is establishing a home support team that can include relatives, friends, neighbors, and yes, even coworkers and employer. These people are your worker bees. I cannot stress enough the importance of establishing a home support team, which is invaluable during the pregnancy and even more so after the birth. Initially, you may feel overwhelmed at just the thought of adding this task to your already hectic life as a new mom, but I assure you that once you put the home support team into action, your life will be less hectic. You will discover a small measure of the team's value as you read through this chapter. I suggest that you discuss with your husband the details of who will be on the team and their responsibilities, and then get the ball rolling.

The first order of business will be for you to acknowledge your husband to act as the primary person of support. He—not your mother, mother-in-law, or anyone else—should be the heart of the support team. You should trust him implicitly. He is the person of first contact with whom you should communicate to make sure the pregnancy runs smoothly with the help of other members of the home team. As I noted in Chapter 1, your husband should come before anyone, including the baby. This is one way of demonstrating your love and faith in him. It also boosts his image as the man and new dad of the family without you losing your identity as a new mom. Without a husband and dad, there will be no new family.

Look at it this way: What happens if you die? Wouldn't you want your husband to be the baby's primary point of contact and advocate? How could he be if you don't acknowledge him during the pregnancy as the primary person on the home team? How would he be prepared to deal with the challenges of being a single parent?

There are only two exceptions in which a husband should not be the primary go-to person for your support team. One is if your husband's work requires travel or long periods of time away from home in a profession such as a doctor, salesman, fireman, police detective, CEO, or military serviceman. If this is the case, you can designate him as co-primary supporter. The second exception is if you ask your husband and he declines. And it is okay for him to say no. He may be too overwhelmed to take on such a role. The point is that you asked him first. If this is the case, then give your husband the courtesy of suggesting the person he'd like to see as the primary person of your home support team. Once you come to a mutual agreement, then continue with the selection process. And if he changes his mind down the road, you should ask the initial person you invited to step aside. (You may want to let the first person know ahead of time about the possible change.)

Before I explain how to select the team members and delegate their responsibilities, I cannot stress enough how important it is to coordinate and manage this home support team during the pregnancy. If you incorporate your home team immediately after the announcement of the pregnancy, you will have about eight months to train and fine-tune your team of worker bees. The sooner you start, the better, because it will take a while for you and your husband to manage the personnel, delegate the responsibilities, and resolve any problems you may encounter. As well-intended as people may be, you don't know how well they will come through for you. If one person flakes out on you, you'll have to replace him or her with someone else you can count on. Or you may want to experiment with having people share a common responsibility to cover yourself in case one person is ill or unavailable because of an emergency in their family.

By the time the baby is born, you'll have an efficient system and team in place to assist you with the caring of the newborn and give you more time to enjoy being a new mom.

After you name your husband as the primary supporter, it is imperative that all members of the home team understand that he is in charge and that any communication or changes regarding the support team's duties should always include him. Do not undermine his position of authority. If you do, the support team will not function properly. Everyone must be on the same page. If anyone (including your mom or his mom) on the team does not cooperate, a consequence should follow. The commitment to your husband as the primary supporter and your commitment to follow through with carrying out consequences is an example of how you can show respect to the title of Dad I discussed in Chapter 8.

Always remember you and your husband are in charge of the pregnancy and decide who does what. If you're gun-shy about inviting or asking people to help, don't be. Trust me, people want to help but can't unless you tell them what you need. As for inviting people to join your team, do not make order of importance an issue. The main goal is to match the duty with a person most competent to complete the task. If you don't, you may find yourself spending more time making up for the person's incompetence and then defeating the whole purpose of this project. However, be careful not to jump the gun if a person doesn't meet your expectations. This is probably a new experience for him or her as well, so exercise a little patience.

The next step is to take an inventory list of duties you and your husband will delegate to your home team. I'm not going to supply you with a long laundry list because each couple will have different priorities for what duties they would like their team members to perform. Duties can include house maintenance and repairs, gardening, car washing, grocery errands, or emergencies like taking a pet to the vet. You may have duties that you are not willing to give up to other people, and that's okay. What is important is that you communicate what you'd like done and how you'd like it done to your satisfaction. But don't go overboard on the expectations, and remember to focus on what people do for you and not how they do it.

Also keep in mind that the home support team is not just about getting stuff done. Their presence alone can provide moral support and great comfort to you and your husband. There may be times when you just need someone to talk to when your husband is not around, and likewise with your husband.

Although it is important to have a home support team at your disposal, you should also recognize the value it will bring to helping your husband be more than just the financial supporter of your new family.

18
It's important for you to respect my male friendships

After a woman and man marry, both express some resentment towards each other's friends. There are husbands who don't take a liking to wives spending time with their friends, especially male friends, and vice versa with the wives. There is also resentment from the friends towards the spouse. These are normal emotions. Regardless of the gender, friends can put a wrinkle into a marriage, especially when the husband and wife become parents.

For a new mom to have continued relationships with female friends is an accepted practice. The same is not true for husbands and their male friends, whom new moms will often resent. Whatever the origins of the jealousy, it is not healthy for the marriage. It's okay to feel jealousy because it is a normal emotion humans feel. (It serves as a defense mechanism.) However, it's important to keep jealousy in check and not allow the green monster to make you feel insecure and like you have to control everything. The problem is often not with the friends per se but the way a wife reacts to or judges them. Some wives feel threatened by their husbands' friends. If a husband is spending time with his friends, he is not spending it with her. Some wives fear one of their husband's friends will have a negative influence on him. Some view most friendships their husbands have as toxic to their marriage. As a result, some wives will carry out a friendship audit to decide who can still be friends with their husbands. Jealousy to this extent is not healthy for a marriage and will only cause more stress and tension, which you don't need during the pregnancy.

The green monster can also place a husband in an uncomfortable predicament. If he doesn't stand up to his wife, he may lose a friend and be labeled as a wimp. If he doesn't stand up to his friend, his marriage will suffer. Barring drug, alcohol, or gambling addiction or inappropriate behavior, a new dad or new mom shouldn't be placed in a position to make a choice between a friend and a spouse. Would you approve of your husband asking you to give marching orders to your girlfriends? I don't think so.

While new moms respect and see the value of having female friends involved in the pregnancy, most new moms do not offer the same courtesy to their husbands' friendships. One example is the ceremonial baby shower party hosted by a female friend for the mom-to-be. The baby shower is a big what-to-do for the dad because most of them are women-only events. Why doesn't our culture consider a party for new dads to celebrate the arrival of the baby and his journey into fatherhood? I sense it has to do with the way our culture distinguishes between bachelorette and bachelor parties.

The bachelor party has been given an unfair and bad reputation, in part because the event is perceived as a rite of passage into marriage that symbolizes the last time the groom is free of his future wife's influence. People immediately envision adolescent, hazing-like pranks at the future groom's expense that can include a seductive female stripper. Not every bachelor party involves a stripper, and for those that do, rarely is the groom involved in any mischievous activity with a stripper, and if he is, more often than not it is done in good fun. (On the flip side, a bachelorette party is not as innocent as one might think. I know. I crashed a bachelorette party once, and some of the hazing the women displayed was just as—if not more—sexually repulsive than what I've witnessed at a bachelor party. And the women also knew how to have their way with the sexy male stripper they hired for entertainment.) As much as a new mom doesn't want to approve of some or all of her husband's friends, she really can't justify asking him to cut off all ties with them.

Remember the golfing scenario I addressed in Chapter 7? Here is the solution to helping your husband keep his friendship alive. If a friend invites a dad to play golf, one option is to play only nine holes instead of eighteen. This is an amicable compromise unless a new dad goes overboard and schedules too many golf outings.

If a new mom can take a moment to not allow the green monster to bring out the worst in her, she might be more apt to accept and see the value of her husband's relationship with his friends and how important they are to his growth as a new dad. While a husband has his own unique genetic traits, friends also play a part in shaping his character. The camaraderie a new dad has cultivated over the years with his friends is important to him. His friends represent the history of his pre-dad life, and now he wants them to be a part of his post-dad life. A new dad doesn't need a wife to play judge and jury. As I noted in Chapter 8 about respect, I'm not asking you to like his friends, just to honor his relationships with his friends.

A new mom already understands the value her girlfriends bring to the pregnancy such as support and comfort. Guess what? A new dad's friends are just as capable if a new mom gives them the opportunity. Don't use the same false perceptions of men as inept dads to prejudge your husband's friends as being bad influences on him. You can turn the cards around and maybe look at how your husband's role as a new dad can have a positive influence on his male friends. Someday one of his single friends will become a new dad, and he'll have the benefit of your husband's guidance based on experiences of his involvement during the pregnancy. Or if one of his friends is a dad, he might offer your husband some great advice because he has been through a pregnancy before. In either case, everybody benefits. And you and your husband benefit the most because now you have more members available to become part of the home support team I discussed in the previous chapter.

Now start planning a party for your husband and his friends and get to know them better.

19
I'm confused about my role as a dad in today's world

During my dad's generation in the 1950s, a dad had one major role to fulfill, and that was as the breadwinner. A dad also played the role of protector and disciplinarian but only when it didn't interfere with his work schedule. Although an unfair assessment, a typical 1950s dad was described as a stoic, workaholic couch potato who relied on his wife to do all the parenting and household chores, and was emotionally distant from his child. Fatherhood was fairly simple. So simple that all a dad had to do during the pregnancy was wait in the delivery room. And the day after the birth, he was back to work earning money to support his new family.

When I decided to become a dad in 1987, fatherhood was a bit more complicated. Unlike my dad, I was expected to be more than just the financial provider, disciplinarian, and protector. There was a lot of pressure to be hands-on and take some of the slack off of the duties once reserved only for a mom. I was expected to take on household chores during the pregnancy that were off-limits to my dad. I was also expected to attend doctor appointments and childbirth classes. And, unlike my dad, I was allowed in the delivery room to witness the birth of our baby.

By the mid 1990s, fatherhood took another dramatic twist with a new culture of fathers who were at-home dads. We were dads who traded our Home Depot tool belt and hammer for an apron and broom. This unconventional style of fathering brought a new meaning to the word fatherhood. Around the same time, another major change occurred. The health-care industry introduced a program called Boot Camp for New Dads (BCND) into hospitals. BCND is a unique father-to-father-based workshop that prepares expectant dads for fatherhood. A very small population of men was now attending a class to learn how to be better, more involved dads.

Today's new dad definitely has to deal with higher expectations and a longer laundry list of dadly duties than previous generations of dads did. But this doesn't mean that 1950s dads weren't involved—they were, but in a different way. The way historians portray dads in that period as emotionally distant and uninvolved is not an accurate portrayal of fatherhood. The world was different back then, and our culture didn't teach or allow new dads to participate in responsibilities expected of today's new dads. Given the circumstances, the dads of yesteryear did an amazing job.

While today's dad has access to more information and resources than the 1950s dad, the world of fatherhood has a set of puzzling principles and mixed messages.

- One minute a husband is recognized as a new dad. The next minute he is referred to as a coach, partner, or significant other.
- One minute a husband follows through with his commitment to be a nurturing dad. The next minute his masculinity is questioned.
- One minute a new dad is asked to spend less time at work and more time at home. The next minute a new dad receives a complaint from his wife that there isn't enough money to pay the bills.
- One minute a new dad's employer professes to have a father-friendly work environment. The next minute the employer makes a new dad feel as if his job is in jeopardy because of his newfound commitment to his family.
- One minute an advertisement points out the importance of a dad in a child's life. The next minute another ad tells a dad he isn't doing enough.
- One minute the media points out the benefit of an involved dad. The next minute the media publishes an article that states women don't need a man to help them raise children.

- One minute an ad announces that dads need to be more involved in the pregnancy. The next minute his needs are ignored or he is ostracized and alienated by people (predominately women) at the doctor's office, hospital, family resource center, and baby supply store.

Motherhood has never been put through the kind of scrutiny that fatherhood has in the last sixty years. Nor have mothers had their femininity questioned. No matter what new dads do, it never seems to be good enough. And no matter how hard they try, they never seem to get it right.

A perfect example is the way moms and our society have reacted to the at-home dad community. Instead of embracing the at-home dads, most moms feel threatened by them. Instead of focusing on the benefits of having an at-home dad in the community, people publicly second-guess his decision and ridicule him with jokes. When an at-home dad decides to return to the workforce and applies for a job, his commitment to his family is held against him.

Another example is how children, when shown a safety video about strangers, are indoctrinated with the notion that men are not to be trusted. Why is the stranger in the video always a man? If a strange woman entered a playground, most people would assume that she was the mother of a child at the playground. If a strange man entered the playground, the first reaction is to be suspicious of him.

With these messages of distrust and discontent about men and fatherhood permeating our society, it is a lot easier for a new dad to be confused about his role during the pregnancy.

As new dads step into and through fatherhood, they also feel like they are walking on eggshells and feel under the microscope 24/7. This makes it difficult for a man to stay on the daddy track, and it dims his outlook for a bright future as a dad. How can he stay on track if every few miles, he is bumped off with unwarranted backhanded comments? Even the Little Engine That Could would have a difficult time reaching the top of the hill if he was constantly de-railed.

There are a lot of hardworking and dedicated men in our society who want to be the best new dad they can be. They are all saying, "I know I can, I know I can, I know I can," but they keep getting blindsided and derailed. I think it is time to show how much we appreciate them and help them stay on the daddy track.

20

I'd like you to honor and embrace my role as the breadwinner

As much as new moms would like to have their husbands more involved in the pregnancy, the reality is that being a breadwinner is in a man's DNA. The ability to earn money is the essence of a new dad's identity and a measurement of his self-worth, just as being pregnant and being a caregiver is for a new mom. When you take away a new dad's self-worth, you take away his dignity. Without his dignity, he loses his desire to become an involved dad. Furthermore, not every new dad can accommodate every new mom's request to be involved during the pregnancy due to the nature of his profession or job.

For most expectant couples, the husband is the primary breadwinner. His earning power provides the essentials like food, clothing, housing, medical, life and auto insurance, and for those lucky enough, some luxuries. The money he earns will also pay for the medical bills and other expenses related to the baby. No expectant couple can survive without money, but somehow, new moms and our society have forgotten this very important economic factor.

The importance of money and the role of the breadwinner cannot be overstated. In addition to providing for his family, the breadwinner's earnings also protect a new family from poverty. Unfortunately, because of the aggressive campaign to persuade dads to be more involved in the pregnancy, new moms and the pregnancy industry have downplayed, discounted, and taken for granted the role of the breadwinner.

Although a new dad pays the bills with his hard-earned money, he receives very little in return for his financial investment. There is ample evidence to show that products and services available for a new mom far outnumber those available for a new dad. Take a good look at how hospitals and businesses like family resource centers, bookstores, and baby accessory stores market their services and products. When it comes to pregnancy (and parenting), the main target market is a woman. Businesses spend millions of dollars advertising to a pregnant or new mother. Why? The rationale is that a new mom spends the money, and she naturally follows suit without a second thought. While a new mom spends money through the pregnancy pipeline like it's growing on trees, she and other people have overlooked that she cannot spend money unless her husband has first earned it.

Working mothers who are the primary breadwinners or earn more than their husbands can certainly relate to the point I'm making here. Ask any working mom who's the primary breadwinner, and I'm sure she'll agree that she not only takes great pride in the role but also feels a sense of independence and greater entitlement to the money because she earned it. Furthermore, she'd like her husband to appreciate every dollar she earns and not take her earned income or role as the breadwinner for granted.

Some dads are stuck between a rock and a hard place when it comes to balancing work and family, making it difficult to devote more time to family. In turn, their duty as breadwinner may be unappreciated by their wives and others.

"I'm the primary breadwinner of the family, and I'm all for being more involved, but my job requires that I travel a lot. I can't be the hands-on dad she and I want me to be, so where does that put me in the grand scheme of things? I pay all the bills. Doesn't that count for anything? Am I a bad dad? I don't think so."

"I'm a doctor and put in long hours. I'd like to be around more for my wife and new baby. But I can't. A lot of people are counting on me to keep their families healthy. And if I lose my job, I lose my ability to be the breadwinner. I don't think it's fair to make me feel like I'm not doing enough as a new dad just because I'm not as involved as other new dads."

"I work the graveyard shift and can't make most of the childbirth classes. Because I'm not there doesn't mean I don't want to be involved or make me a bad dad because I'm not involved. But my wife and relatives sure are making me feel that way."

"I work for the FBI in a special counter intelligence unit. I'm on call 24/7 to serve my country. Of course I want to be there for her, but in my profession, duty to country comes first. I can't always be there for my wife and she knows it."

"I'm a commercial fisherman and gone for long periods of time. What I earn puts food on the table and pays the bills."

For those dads who have more flexibility at work, there are choices available to them they may not be aware of. Remember the dad's dilemma I shared with you in Chapter 7? Here is a possible solution.

1. Have your husband approach coworkers and ask some of them to temporarily take some of the slack at the office. (Someday he may be able to return the favor.)
2. Once the coworkers agree, outline a game plan on paper for your employer, schedule a meeting, and submit it to him. Most employers will appreciate the proactive approach in handling this work-life balance issue and then accommodate the new dad.

3. Since your husband will be scaling back on his work, it could result in less pay, especially if part of his income relies on commission. This means a new mom will have to accept a change in lifestyle and restructure the family's budget.

If all parties agree to this arrangement, a new mom can show how much she appreciates her husband by sticking to the new budget and sending a thank-you card to the employer and coworkers for their cooperation. Of course, this is the ideal arrangement. However, it is good to consider other options if there is no cooperation from the employer or coworkers.

If this arrangement cannot be worked out, a new mom has two other options. One is to make the best of the situation and appreciate whatever time a new dad can give. Second is to discuss the idea of her husband finding another company to work for or another career. The reality is that in most cases, a new mom cannot have the best of both worlds.

Regardless of whether a new dad wants to or cannot spend more time with his wife during the pregnancy, a new dad would like a wife to show her appreciation for the hard work he puts into being the breadwinner. And more often than not, compromises have to and can be made. Since a new dad can't be in two places at one time, there has to be a game plan with a little bit of give-and-take, one that will work best for your family.

21
I'd like you to help people respect my role as a new dad

If a man insulted another man's wife, almost every husband would speak up and defend his wife's honor. This gallant act is what a woman expects from a man because chivalry is part of the natural order of manhood and one of many ways a man proves his love for a woman. Chivalry is often used to describe courteous behavior of a man towards a woman. And when a man does come to the aid of a woman, most women appreciate their noble deed.

But what is the protocol for a woman when another person insults her husband and the dad-to-be of her child? There doesn't seem to be one, but there should be, especially in today's world of sexual equality. I believe the major reason there isn't a modus operandi for women is that there is a tendency for courtesies from a woman to a man to be viewed less favorably than those courtesies from a man to a woman. I feel a woman can be chivalrous in a Joan-of-Arc way without making her husband look bad. In this age of sexual equality, isn't it sexist to think that only women can be the objects of chivalry and not be chivalrous? If a woman can stand up for sexual equality, she should also be able to stand up for her husband when he is being treated unfairly. But as the following comments by dads show, most wives don't.

"One of my wife's girlfriends made a statement about how men are so inept at being dads. I was waiting for my wife to voice her support for me because she knew how much I've done for her during the pregnancy. Instead, she let her girlfriend continue with the dad bashing."

"My wife told me that her girlfriend, who is already a mom, was hemming and hawing about her husband Dan's lack of involvement with the baby. I asked why she was telling me this. She said because she was concerned that I may become like Dan. I asked my wife if she said anything to her girlfriend to support that I wouldn't turn out like Dan. She said no."

"My mother-in-law made a backhanded comment about me. She thought I was too involved in the pregnancy and should give my wife some space of her own.

Of course, my wife didn't stand up for me because she didn't want to hurt her mom's feelings. Well, what about my feelings and telling her mom how much she appreciates the stuff I do around the house?"

"My in-laws suggested that I needed to seek another profession so I could earn more money to provide for my new family. My wife and I are happy with our arrangement. But when it came time to stand up to her parents, she had nothing to say."

"After we told both our parents that I would be the at-home parent, they all balked at the idea. Although my wife and I made the decision together, she didn't voice her support for me when it really counted."

"I told the childbirth instructor how I didn't appreciate being referred to as the coach. She didn't seem to care. Then I told my wife and she thought I was making a mountain out of a molehill."

"I had made arrangements with my employer to take four weeks off after the baby's birth so I could be more involved and help my wife out. Two weeks before the due date, my wife said she was going to spend the first five days at her mom's house. Why didn't my wife stand up to her mom and tell her that she wanted to be home with me?"

There are other examples throughout this book that demonstrate how a dad's perspective is given no credibility, how his needs are not addressed, and how the female-dominated world of pregnancy discriminates against dads in much the same way corporate America once did against women. Yet women continue to be gun-shy about speaking up on a dad's behalf.

When these incidents occur, it is imperative that a new mom speak up immediately. A new dad needs to know his wife is willing to go to bat for him in the heat of the moment. Not three, four, or five days or even weeks later. However, if you feel uncomfortable in a face-to-face situation, it's okay to address the person who has offended him by phone or letter within a day, but let your husband know about it.

Sadly, if a new dad did speak up, he would come across as a whiner. But he is not whining. He is only sharing how he feels about the way he was treated. When a new mom doesn't acknowledge a new dad's feelings or voice her support for him, her lack of attention to address the matter will lead to his lack of desire to be involved during the pregnancy.

When a man's opinion falls on deaf ears, there is only one thing left to do: hide in his man cave. If you don't want your husband to seek refuge in his man cave, then speak up.

A new dad is already at a disadvantage because of limited resources and support. A mom's voice carries a lot of weight and can have a major influence in making immediate changes. When you notice any discrepancies in what someone tells you regarding dads or your husband points them out, don't be afraid to write a letter and advocate on his behalf. If a new mom really wants her husband to be a hands-on new dad, then she'll have to demonstrate it by publicly voicing her support for him. I implore you to find the courage to speak up for your husband just as you would like him to do for you.

To stress the importance of advocating for your husband, fast-forward twenty-five years. Your son is now a dad-to-be or your daughter is a mom-to-be. If you want your son or son-in-law to be better prepared for fatherhood and have access to products, services, and resources to help him succeed as a new dad, then speak up now!

22
I'd like you to value my thoughts about the delivery room

Up until the 1970s, dads weren't allowed in the deliver room. In 1974, thanks to Dr. Robert Bradley, founder of the Bradley method of natural childbirth, hospitals opened the delivery room doors for dads to be present during the birth. Since then new moms expect their husbands to be in the delivery room, as this adaptation of Shakespeare's Hamlet soliloquy demonstrates.

> To be or not to be in the delivery room; that is the question.
> Whether 'tis nobler in the mind to suffer
> The pain and blood of a miraculous, wondrous event
> Or to take arms against a sea of anxieties
> And by opposing them? To enjoy; to appreciate.

Shakespeare's play about Hamlet's musing over the pain of life and fear of the uncertainty of death is not unlike a new dad's ambivalence towards the delivery room. Like Hamlet's uncertainties, the unknown and uncertainty of what the delivery room will bring torments a new dad, even though he knows the end result will bring him joy.

Although it is natural for a mom to feel she should take ownership of the delivery room just as she does the baby (as noted in Chapter 3), the fact that she is the one who is pregnant doesn't grant or entitle her to designate herself as the decision maker. Remember, your husband is an equal partner, and as I noted in the Introduction, all a husband wants is his voice to be heard and acknowledged. Therefore, it is important for a new mom to value and consider his thoughts and concerns and include him in the decision-making process.

Oftentimes a new dad is made to feel that he needs to submit to his wife's decisions, and even if he disagrees, he needs to suck it up and support her. But not every new dad embraces the idea to witness the birth for legitimate reasons and would prefer to pass the time in the comfort of a waiting room. Eight months of anticipation creates a lot of anxiety in a new dad. Some of the fears include:

1. Feeling squeamish at the sight of his wife being in pain and at the sight of blood
2. Fear of fainting and distracting the medical staff from caring for his wife and baby

3. Fear of accidentally knocking down a piece of equipment

4. Fear that watching the birth may have a negative effect on his intimate relationship with his wife and lead to sexual dysfunction

5. Fear that something may go wrong

6. Fear his presence may compromise the safety of his wife and baby

In addition to fears, a new dad will also struggle with his role as Dad in the delivery room. This is why it is so important for the childbirth instructors to stop referring to a dad as a coach, cheerleader, assistant, or significant other. A husband needs to know that he is the dad and therefore the primary supporter and advocate. He is your second set of eyes and the person who is there to make sure everything goes according to plan.

Another concern is the new dad managing his time in the delivery room. Most couples like to take photos or videotape the birth. Juggling the role of director, photographer, and cameraman can be very taxing for a new dad. If he is caught up in all the hoopla of a Hollywood production of the birth, he may not have time to enjoy the experience as a dad. An alternative is to invite a relative or friend or hire a person to videotape and photograph the birth. If you choose to do this, you will give up some privacy. Either way, the important thing is that you include him in part of the decision process, respect his feelings, and come to a mutual agreement.

The bottom line is that whatever issues your husband has about the delivery room, give his perspective the credibility it deserves.

23

I don't want you to be the "perfect" pregnant mom

We all know that there is no such thing as a "perfect" person. Yet most new moms have become obsessed with perfection and have bought into romanticizing unrealistic expectations of being the "perfect" pregnant mom. Who created this mythical creature? How and where did the hype start?

First let me tell you who didn't create the myth: husbands. Most husbands know there is no such thing as a "perfect" wife, so the pressure to be a "perfect" pregnant mom didn't come from men. Most dads I know will also tell you that "Super Moms" make lousy wives. If a wife puts too much effort at any time into being "Super Mom," how can she have any time left to be a wife?

According to Susan Douglas and Meredith Michaels,

coauthors of *The Mommy Myth: The Idealization of Mother-hood and How It Has Undermined Women,* the media has played a huge role in pressuring and brainwashing new moms to be perfect. Douglas and Michaels analyzed the past thirty years of media images about mothers: the superficial achievements of the celebrity mom, the staging of the "mommy wars" between working mothers and stay-at-home moms, and the onslaught of values-based marketing that raises mothering standards to impossible levels.

Another factor that has contributed to the creation of the mythical "perfect" mom is what I noted in Chapter 8. Because new moms have been indoctrinated with the false notion of men being inept as dads, they feel obligated to make up for their husbands' unwarranted inadequacies as new dads. One of the most common responses a new dad receives from his wife after she shares her frustration about him not completing a chore or task to her satisfaction is "Never mind, I'll do it myself. Why do I have to do everything?"

A husband would like to say to his wife, "You don't. And I don't expect you to do it all." But doing so may land him in the doghouse.

Moms must also take some responsibility for creating this unrealistic goal of perfection because they have bought into values-based marketing and turned motherhood into a competition. Businesses, including hospitals, have turned pregnancy into a billion-dollar industry. They target the emotions of new moms to generate sales of their products and services and bombard them with junk mail and promotions. *If you really want to be the "perfect" pregnant mom,* they imply, *you need this, this, this, and that.* The next thing you know, a new mom winds up competing against other moms to be "perfect" or "more perfect" by purchasing items and services they really don't need. The gratification of just being a new mom is not enough anymore, and now she needs material things to build her self-esteem and make her feel like a "perfect" mom. While a new mom is caught up in this buying binge, she is wasting money and often running up a huge amount of debt. This is another reason a husband doesn't want his wife to try to be the "perfect" pregnant mom.

Before the pregnancy there wasn't enough time in a twenty-four-hour day to be a "perfect" wife. So it's unrealistic for a new mom to think she can add more responsibilities to her already hectic schedule and still be "perfect."

If a new mom is doing everything to be "perfect," how can she expect her husband, as well as the people on her home support team, to learn how to do anything for her? If a new mom also gives the impression that she doesn't need help because she is "perfect," people will really think she doesn't need help. The truth is that you and your husband really do need help. If a new mom can't control herself from trying to be a "perfect" pregnant mom, imagine how much more pressure she'll place on herself after the birth of the baby.

So why do most new moms have trouble letting go of

this need to be a "perfect" pregnant mom? It's the pleasing-and-guilt gene. New moms are under the impression that to be "perfect," they have to please everybody, even at the expense of alienating their husbands. And if they don't please, they feel guilty.

New moms need to say "no" more often to marketers and people who make them feel like they need another product or service. And they need to say "yes" more often when people offer or ask them whether they need help. As one husband said, "Why is it so easy for my wife to say no to me when I ask for sex? But she can't say no to a salesperson who encourages her to buy an item or service she really doesn't need."

The need to do everything is also a control issue. Relinquishing a task or chore can be difficult for a new mom, but not impossible. Saying "yes" doesn't just mean a new mom is giving a person permission to help—she is also relinquishing control over how the chore or task will be done. A new mom's job is not to inspect the work offered by other people but to appreciate it.

A new mom doesn't have to succumb to the pressure of being the "perfect" pregnant mom when it comes to weight gain. The reality is that you will experience weight gain for obvious reasons. Most new dads don't care about the weight gain or your appearance because they understand it's temporary. Some new dads even find a pregnant woman sensuous. You will also experience lack of energy, less time to get things done, challenges and issues you can't resolve alone, and imperfection. These experiences are normal and unavoidable, so stop beating yourself up, because a new mom cannot do it all.

The key is to stay in the real world. *Perfection* is a dirty word and a fantasy that will only lead to guilt and disappointment. You don't have to buy every product or service offered to you. You don't have to let the media and other people define or measure your success as a mother. It is healthy to strive for excellence in being a new mom, but not for perfection.

I don't know any person who has attained perfection. Do you?

Working to always be perfect is exhausting. And the truth is that no matter how hard a person tries to be perfect, there will always be room for improvement.

The way a new dad sees it is that the less a new mom worries about being perfect, the more time she has to focus on keeping herself and the baby healthy, but more important, time to enjoy being a new mom.

24

I have fears about becoming a dad

Every new dad and mom have some level of fear about bringing a human being into the world. It is a life-changing experience and carries with it a lot of responsibility. Fear is a natural, instinctual response and plays an important role in our daily lives. This emotion is programmed into our brains as a safety mechanism to help increase our chances of survival.

Fear is an emotion people don't often talk about because they don't want to admit they're scared. This is especially true with men. But that doesn't mean women aren't scared about becoming moms. They are. The level of fear a new dad experiences, however, is much greater than a new mom's if she takes advantage of the wealth of information, services, and resources available to her. With a comprehensive support system in place, a new mom's fear diminishes quickly, and she is able to continue with less anxiety. Every step of the way she is given assurance that she will overcome her fear of being a new mom. A new dad doesn't have this luxury.

Everyone has some level of fear. It's just as hard for a man to admit he is wr . . . wr . . . wr . . . not right as it is to admit he is scared. Some new dads handle it better than others. The truth is that most men don't handle fear very well, not because they don't know how, but rather because of their egos and the reactions they receive from their male friends. Ironically, a man is more afraid of what other people, especially male peers, will think than he is of the idea causing the fear. If he were to admit he was scared, he'd be told to suck it up and take it like a man. If he didn't, his masculinity would be questioned. A woman, on the other hand, would receive a different and more compassionate response.

Some new dads will tell you that they don't have any fears, but they're in total denial. Some of the fears I have already covered, like anxiety about not being a wife's main squeeze, the health of baby and mom, hurting the baby, and finances. But a new dad also has other fears on his mind.

One of them is wondering what kind of father he will be. A new dad is concerned about the effect his upbringing will have on him. While a new dad's childhood environment and family dynamics do play a part, they are not the determining factor. I know good dads who survived an abusive and/or emotionally absent father. I know good dads who were raised by a single working mother or father. I know good dads who had no father in their lives due to an early death. And I know absent and dysfunctional dads who had a good father as a role model. My life as a child falls into the first two categories. However, I had the good fortune of being reunited with my father before I became a new dad.

What most dads fail to recognize is that regardless of how a new dad was raised, nobody can predict how good or bad any man will be as a father.

I will acknowledge that growing up in a functional family increases a new dad's ability to become a good dad. But there is no guarantee because there are too many variables that can knock a man off the daddy track. Just because a new dad's father was the perfect role model doesn't ensure he'll be the same. And just because a new dad's father was dysfunctional doesn't mean he'll be dysfunctional.

"My father was abusive and never around. I didn't have a good role model. So I feel I'm going into fatherhood totally unprepared, and that scares me."

"I was raised by a single working mom. I'm not scared of becoming a dad. I'm petrified!"

"My dad cheated on my mother. I'm not only worried about what kind of dad I will be, I'm also worried about what kind of husband I will be. Will I give into temptation like my dad?"

"My dad was a workaholic and alcoholic. I don't want to be like him."

"Am I really ready to be a dad? There is so much I don't know about being one."

"My dad was a great father. He was devoted to my mom and helped her with the household chores. It is going to be tough to fill his shoes."

Regardless of the circumstances, the pressure to be a good dad is intense. Even a dad who grew up with a good role model has to deal with the stress and high expectations of filling his father's shoes.

Another fear a dad may have is of mortality. As I mentioned earlier, a new dad will have anxieties about his wife and baby surviving the birth. Questions that run through his mind include, *If the baby dies, how will I handle the loss with my wife? If my wife dies, how will I live without her? What will happen if I get in a car accident? If I'm disabled, how will I provide for my new family? If I die, what will happen to my wife and child?*

Whether you're a dad or a mom, fear is okay. Don't let your husband lose sleep over the fear. Instead, help him view fear as a wake-up call to the serious nature of the journey he is about to take. Only time will tell whether he will become a good dad. Hopefully, he'll rise to the occasion and turn into the dad you dreamed he would be.

25

I may need your help making peace with my father

Strained father-son relationships can occur even under the best of circumstances within a family and healthy environment. There is no guarantee that every father-son relationship will be harmonious. Unfortunately, bitter rifts that may occur can last a lifetime and never be resolved. What is even more unfortunate is that the collateral damage passes from one generation to the next—all because neither side is willing to make peace. But there is something today's new dads can do to stop the cycle. As I noted in my book *Pacifi(her): What She's Thinking When She's Pregnant,* "There is a choice you have to make in everything you do. And you must always keep in mind the choice you make, makes you."

Since it's tough to teach an old dog new tricks, I feel it is up to the son to swallow his pride and make the first step into healing the emotional wound that exists between father and son. A son should extend this courtesy to a dad out of respect for him and also view it as a way to make peace with himself to prevent any burden of guilt he might feel if he didn't make an effort to repair the relationship.

In the open-discussion workshops I facilitate for new dads, I invite them to talk about their fathers during the introduction. The purpose of this exercise is to empower today's new dad to heal an old wound and to recognize that he can't move forward to accomplish his goal of not turning out like his dad until he makes peace with his father. Please note that I'm not necessarily advocating that a new dad completely repair his relationship with his father, because some relationships just aren't repairable. Knowing that he made the effort is all that matters for a new dad. Once the ball is in his father's court, there is not much more the new dad can do to repair the strained relationship.

Most new dads balk at the idea of openly discussing such a personal and intimate topic, especially in front of a group of strangers. But I set the dads at ease by assuring them that the purpose of this exercise is not to put their dads on trial. When my dad was a father, he did what he was taught and told to do by our culture. His primary role was to be the breadwinner. He wasn't expected to attend doctor's appointments and was not allowed in the delivery room. After the birth, he never even changed a diaper and was never allowed to be alone with me.

While the next generation of dads was more hands-on, our culture was still not very accepting of the new "involved" role they were beginning to play. Yes, dads attended doctor's visits and were allowed in the delivery room, but as I've previously mentioned, the environment wasn't and still isn't father-friendly. Yes, dads change diapers, but most moms hesitate to allow—or will not allow—their husbands to be alone with the baby. How many moms do you know who would leave a baby alone with a dad with the same level of trust she would have leaving it with another mom? Not many.

I honestly believe most of the past generations of dads did want to be hands-on fathers. Unfortunately, our culture prevented and deprived them from taking a leap of faith into becoming involved dads. If you don't believe me, take a look at how our culture treats at-home dads. Most people still don't like the idea of a man coming into the pantry and being the primary caregiver.

There is no quick fix to heal an emotional wound that has grown for years from an absentee father. And burying the pain is unhealthy. Taking the first step in healing an estranged father-son relationship will not be easy for your husband, and of course it will be very painful, but he'll be a better man for it. One way to help your husband take this leap of faith is to reassure him that he—not his father—has control over whether reconciliation will cause more rejection, abuse, or pain.

A new dad's efforts may not result in the desired out-
come of a blissful father-son relationship, but that's okay.
Remember, this isn't about how a father responds to his
son's efforts. Whether a new dad wants forgiveness from his
father or wants to forgive his father is up to him. It all boils
down to the son making peace with himself, not with his
dad.

But how does a new dad reconcile with his biological
father if he isn't around or can't be found? Although there
are lots of questions a new dad would like answered and
emotions he'd like to share, the only remedy may be to accept that reconciliation will be found only by making peace
within himself.

Regardless of the painful baggage, at the end of the day,
only a new dad has the power to break the dysfunctional-
dad cycle. Although a new dad's father may not have left
him much of a fatherhood blueprint to follow, a new dad
can leave one for his child.

If your husband had a good father, that is great. But if
your husband didn't, tell him he deserves to be a better dad
than his absentee, dysfunctional father.

26
I also have guilt trips

During the open-discussion groups I conduct for expectant dads, I ask them to submit a fathering issue they would like to have the group address. After several years, I thought I had collected a complete list of all the issues a new dad faced. But during one group session, a courageous new dad proved me wrong.

"Hogan, I've got an issue I'd like to address."

"What is it, Ryan?"

"Guilt."

Ryan caught me off guard because I never thought about guilt as an issue for dads, including myself, because the word is always associated with pregnant women. Guilt is such a huge issue for a new mom that most feel guilty for feeling guilty. Even when a mom feels she deserves to pamper herself, after she does, she feels guilty about her decision. So I had to ask him to share his thoughts about the guilt he felt.

"I have to admit that this is a first," I said. "I'm not sure I understand what you mean by guilt. Can you describe what you're feeling guilty about?"

"Yes, I feel guilty about not being able to provide enough money or spend time with my wife and new baby. I'm already working overtime now to pay for the bills. I also feel guilty because my work schedule may not allow me to be there for my wife and baby after the birth as much as I'd like to be."

After Ryan finished, a couple of the dads expressed the same sentiments he had about guilt. What the dads shared with me was a real eye-opener. In retrospect, I realize that I also felt guilt during my early days as a dad. Unfortunately, I didn't have the knowledge or wherewithal to openly address the guilt. Can you imagine people's responses to me if I had brought it up back then? Even today, a man's guilt is not a topic addressed or written about in media publications.

In my research I found a long list of articles and forums about a mom's guilt. Some of the titles included "Kiss Mommy Guilt Goodbye," "31 Reasons You Shouldn't Feel Mom Guilt," "Don't Make Mothers Feel Guilty for Choosing Bottle over Breast," and "Feeling Guilty About Being a Working Mom." However, I had a very difficult time finding reference material about a dad's guilt. What I did find was a remark and question submitted by a new dad at both of these Web sites, www.greatdad.com and www.babycenter. com. The dad explained that he and his wife enjoyed being parents, but that whenever he tried to get extra work done at home, he would feel guilty that he was not doing enough to help out. "I feel guilty about leaving my wife to take care of our child since she's with him all day, and I know she would appreciate a break. I try to help, but I also need to get ahead with work. What should I do?"

It's true that new moms feel a lot of guilt. A recent survey from *Working Mother* magazine found that 57 percent of working mothers feel guilty every single day, and 31 percent feel guilty at least once a week. In the *ParentDish* article "Feeling Guilty About Being a Working Mom" written by Lesley Kennedy, she noted, "There are times when we feel guilty about ten times a day." Of course, there is no research about working dads feeling guilty. If a survey were conducted, I believe the percentages would be lower. But just because a dad may not feel guilt to the same extent and at the same intensity that a mom does doesn't mean that a man doesn't feel guilty at all or shouldn't talk about it.

Our culture is so disconnected when it comes to a working dad feeling guilty that we have yet to address or write articles about it. Yet plenty of published articles have been written for working moms about the guilt they feel. Regardless, the number one guilt is the same for working dads: not being home for their children and spouses. Other guilty feelings dads may have include those addressed by these men.

"I feel bad that I didn't deposit more money in our savings account. I should have prepared better financially."

"I feel bad that I don't have a better job with health benefits. I also feel like I should have gone into a profession that earned more money."

"I wish I could do more to and spend more time to be with and help my wife but I can't because of my military career."

"I wish I could attend more of my wife's doctor's appointments, but I can't because of my business travel schedule. It's tough to be with her when I have to be in China."

"I feel bad that I can drink alcohol and my wife can't."

"I know it's normal to feel resentment towards the baby, but I feel bad when I do."

"I feel bad that I don't have enough patience for my wife's mood swings, especially after I raise my voice and get angry."

Thank goodness Ryan had the courage to speak up. Without him I wouldn't have been able to bring this topic the attention it deserves.

27

I worry about the baby's and your health

One of the top suggestions I hear veteran dads propose to expectant dads is to prepare for the unexpected. It's good advice. But life is so unpredictable that no matter how well a person prepares, he or she can be at the mercy of an unintended consequence or an unexpected turn of events and is oftentimes blindsided. This is especially true with respect to mortality. The grim reality is death can happen during a birth. Death is imminent, yet people are rarely prepared to talk about or deal with the subsequent loss and mourning. Birth is also imminent. Although most births have a happy ending, some do not.

Most new dads understand that the odds of a successful birth resulting in a healthy mom and baby is in their favor. Statistics back this assumption up. According to the

National Center for Health Statistics, 13 infants in 100,000 die from birth, and 679 women per 100,000 die from giving birth. These statistics don't include miscarriages. So that means a total of 520 infants die each year immediately following birth. If we include the deaths of women out of the four million births, which we should because they are directly related to each other, the total is 28,400. Unfortunately the research also shows that women are dying during and after the birth at the highest rate in decades. Experts believe the increase is a result of maternal obesity, older moms, and increased C-sections. Still, the probability of death is relatively low, but a new dad still worries about his wife's and baby's mortality. Although the probability may only dwell in his subconscious, it can lead to increased anxiety.

A new dad's anxiety can begin with worrying about complications that might lead to his wife's and child's death, such as loss of blood, blood poisoning, infection, strangulation from the umbilical cord, and hemorrhaging, followed by emotional and financial hardship. *How will I cope with the news from the doctor? How will I cope with the loss of my wife? How will I cope when sharing the news with relatives and friends? How will I raise our baby without my wife? How will I financially provide for the baby without my wife's help or income? I can't be at home and work at the same time.*

If the baby dies, how will I cope with my wife's loss? How will I cope with my loss? How will it affect our marriage? Will my wife want to become pregnant again? And if my wife and baby die, how will I cope with their loss and life without them?

In addition to worrying about death, a new dad will also worry about the possibility of a deformed or disabled baby. The American College of Obstetricians and Gynecologists estimates that in every 33 babies, 1 baby is born with a birth defect. Birth defects could be due to genetic, hereditary, environmental, or unknown factors. However, even if a baby is born healthy, some babies—as was the case with our middle son, Wesley—may not be diagnosed until sometime after the birth.

Giving birth to a disabled baby brings about a whole different list of anxieties and can even be more devastating than death because there is no closure. With a disabled baby, a new dad inherits a costly medical bill and possibly the huge responsibility of 24/7 care. A baby with a disability also exacerbates the parenting issues and increases the chance of divorce. But the biggest anxiety is losing dreams of life with a healthy child.

Although the odds are that neither of these scenarios will play out in your life, it's a good idea to discuss the *what-ifs* with your husband. If your husband is resistant, don't give up on this issue. But be careful how you deliver your request. I suggest you present the topic in little sound bites. With respect to death, a good way to bring this up is to talk to your husband about your will or living trust. If you don't have one, this is a good time to talk about it. "Honey, I'm not trying to be a worrywart, but I'd like to review our will and talk about what decisions to make in case something tragic happens during the birth." Notice that I didn't mention the words *die* or *death*.

Once you and your husband have broken the ice, the two of you can open up discussions about how to plan his life without you and/or the baby. This is a time to reassure him how much you love him and encourage him that in case of a tragedy, to not feel guilty and move on with his life. Let him know that if you die and the baby lives, you have the utmost confidence in him to be a great dad. Part of the game plan should also include a list of people he can turn to for support. They can be the same people on your home support team. You may also want to think about discussing what to do if he dies or becomes disabled. As I noted in Chapter 24, a new dad will also have anxieties about his own mortality and how you and the baby will survive without him, so it is good to have a game plan for this possible scenario, as well.

The purpose of this exercise is not to just prepare for the unexpected but also to plan for the unexpected. By openly discussing mortality, both of you will have peace of mind knowing that you did everything you could to prepare each other to handle and overcome the unexpected.

28
I need your help balancing time at work and home

For the last twenty years, there has been an aggressive national campaign to encourage dads to spend more time with their wives during the pregnancy. This entails spending less time at work, more time at home, and more time helping with household chores and other responsibilities related to the pregnancy. Most of today's new dads have accepted the invitation and want to be more hands-on than their fathers were. However, one major obstacle that stood in the way of their fathers still exists today. And that is how to find the right balance.

The first question that comes to mind is "How will it be possible to please my employer and wife at the same time?" A new dad can't. It's impossible to deliver one hundred percent satisfaction to both. Unfortunately, that is what an employer and new mom expect from a new dad. Despite the circumstances, a new dad's employer still demands excellence at work and has high expectations, and likewise with a new mom. A new dad suddenly feels more time-pressured. "I already had a hard time juggling a career and married life before the pregnancy. And now I have to squeeze in time to be an involved dad? I'm overwhelmed."

So how do a new dad and mom balance time between careers and parenthood when they are already strapped for time? It will take a collaborative game plan and some flexibility. Unfortunately, although companies profess to be family-friendly, they don't do much to accommodate a new dad or mom. And the services they offer don't really allow a new dad to be hands-on in the way he needs to be. The research also shows that most new dads will not utilize the current family-friendly company policies and services like the Family Medical Leave Act (FMLA) because they fear losing a promotion or their job by putting family first. (Even some of today's working women fear they may lose a promotion or their job if they decide to become pregnant.) What a new dad really needs from his employer is personal time.

There was a time when an expectant mom couldn't relate to the struggles a new dad faced regarding this very challenging issue. And many probably still don't. But today there is a population of working moms who can fully empathize with a working dad's struggle to balance time between his career and fatherhood. In addition to nurturing a marriage and family, today's new mom is also expected to nurture a successful professional career. If you are one of these moms, you will probably nod your head in affirmation. If you're a mom who plans to stay home temporarily or full time, I hope this chapter will shed some light on the importance of collaborating and being flexible with your husband in coming to terms with the best possible game plan that works for your new family.

There is no one-size-fits-all balancing program that will meet the needs of every family because each new family's dynamics are unique. For example, a traveling salesman, doctor, or detective may not have the flexibility or time to be as involved as a UPS employee, bank teller, teacher, or other employee with a regular forty-hour weekday schedule. Therefore, a game plan you create for your family will not necessarily succeed for another family.

The two factors that will determine how to create a game plan for your family are the new dad's career or profession and the relationship with his employer. A part of the game plan may also be predicated on an expectant couple's financial situation, which I covered in Chapter 13. If a couple's financial status is in dire straits, then it will limit their flexibility. For example, a new dad may need to work overtime or two jobs to sustain an income level he needs to provide for his new family. In this case, a new mom will have to either be much more flexible or carry a greater burden of the responsibilities. If your situation is the latter, then it is even more important to establish a home support network as discussed in Chapter 17.

The first order of business is to block a sufficient amount of time to discuss and develop a work-home game plan. This is a serious matter, so give it some serious time. I recommend that your husband take two vacation days off from work—Friday and Monday—and that you use this four-day weekend as a brainstorming session with him, making time for a date night on Saturday evening.

So what should you discuss with your husband?

- Your specific needs, not wants, and realistic expectations
- How much time he is capable of taking off from work
- Whether he needs downtime after he returns home from work
- How much responsibility he is willing to take on at home
- His relationship with his employer
- How much flexibility he has with work
- What personal time of his own he is willing to give up
- A list of responsibilities and chores
- Work options with employers like telecommuting, flextime schedule, or changing shifts
- How to prioritize the list once you establish it
- Changing careers or jobs to something with a more family-friendly environment
- Designating a block of alone time (See Chapter 29)
- Scheduling a time to reevaluate the game plan and possibly make some changes

- A commitment to follow through with the game plan
- A list of consequences for not following through

Once you've established an agreed-upon game plan, do not overwhelm him with a long "honey-do" list. Wean him into the list of chores and new schedule. For the next two weeks, make a trial run of your plan to work out some of the kinks. Begin by giving him three tasks to see how he handles them. Give him an opportunity to delegate a task to one of the home-support-team members. Once he feels comfortable, ask him if he is ready to tackle one or two more requests. The more specific you are, the better he'll be able to follow through. Remember that even with a good game plan, things you never thought of may come up, so be prepared to be flexible and make some adjustments.

Here is an example of what I mean about being flexible. If having your husband attend a doctor's appointment is important to you, then you may have to give up something else on the list like helping out with a household chore. And vice versa.

Remember the domino-effect scenario I presented in Chapter 7? Here is one solution that exemplifies how to utilize the aforementioned list.

A new dad should approach his coworkers and ask how many of them will cover for him at work so he can spend more time with his pregnant wife. (Someday maybe he'll be able to return the favor.) Then he should present the game plan he and his wife discussed to his employer and assure the head honcho that his life as a new dad will not affect his performance at work.

Another example is for a new dad to request to his employer that he take two to four weeks off after the baby's birth by utilizing the FMLA or vacation time. I highly recommend this staycation for every new dad because of the following benefits. First, this gives you a significant amount of time to bond with your new family and help you focus on the job you have ahead of you as a dad. Second, you'll get a chance to hone your skills as a caregiver. Third, you'll develop empathy for your wife in her new role as a mother. Fourth, it will give time for you and your wife to learn how to work together as a team.

By working together and having some flexibility, a new mom and dad can find a balanced lifestyle that will work best for their new family.

29

I need to have some reasonable "me" time

Most new moms undervalue the importance of "me" time. They also view it as a selfish act and oftentimes allow guilt to stand in the way of a well-deserved break from motherhood. This explains why a new mom quarrels with her husband when he decides to take a break from fatherhood.

Most new dads, however, have no qualms or guilt about indulging in some "me" time. They relish what little time is available to participate in a pleasurable activity unrelated to the pregnancy. This lack of guilt explains why a new mom puts up a fuss when a new dad runs off to have a little leisure time by himself or with his buddies.

The truth is that pregnancy is very demanding, so new dads and moms should make time to relieve stress and relax. A new dad may be overwhelmed with his new role and need a break to clear his head and regroup. He will also need the "me" time to avoid burnout and enjoy some freedom from the daily grind of fatherhood that includes attending a doctor's appointment, completing household chores, or caring for his wife, as well as the anxieties and pressures related to finances, health of baby, wife's mood swings, work, and being a new dad.

If a new dad is tired, he is bound to make mistakes and will need time to recharge his batteries. This is also especially true with a new mom because she is using up a lot of energy to feed and nourish two bodies. Not taking a well-deserved break can place her and the baby at risk. Everybody deserves some *reasonable* "me" time and a little freedom. A new mom and dad can even have simultaneous "me" time—there is no reason you can't enjoy quality "me" time while he is enjoying his furlough.

Just because a new mom won't capitalize on "me" time doesn't mean she should prevent her husband from taking some *reasonable* "me" time. The reason I stress *reasonable* is because there are some unreasonable, time-consuming activities a new dad shouldn't be allowed to participate in, like eighteen holes of golf, weekly softball or bowling leagues, or a trip to Vegas. However, if a new dad wants to be a substitute for one or two softball games or bowling matches, I find that to be reasonable.

Reasonable "me" time can include a poker game, drinks

with the boys (if he finds a way to return home safely), a tennis match, a handball match, a pick-up basketball game, skeet shooting, fishing, or a personal hobby. "Me" time can also be spent by himself taking a walk in the woods or on the beach, reading a book, working out at the health club, watching television, or taking a nap.

When a new dad is allowed to spend "me" time unwinding and laughing, he'll usually return home a much happier and more energized man. And who knows, maybe he'll experience a guilt trip along the way and feel motivated to do more work for you around the house.

Now that you have a clear definition of *reasonable* "me" time, here is a list of *don'ts* for new moms.

- Don't make assumptions or think the worst about what he will do during his free time.
- Don't extort the "me" time. Whether a new dad deserves "me" time shouldn't be determined by his performance or lack thereof. He may be tired and need a break to re-energize. A break in the daddy routine is a good thing.
- Don't be the jealous and possessive mom who deliberately prevents her husband from having some free time.
- Don't be a new mom who holds his desire to have "me" time against him.
- Don't keep a choke hold on your husband. It will only discourage him from helping you during the pregnancy.
- Don't keep score. Because of the very nature of you being pregnant, he will have more opportunities for "me"

time than you will. He doesn't have to deal with the discomfort of carrying the baby. And if he is more active and has more friends, he'll probably need more "me" time moments than you.

- Don't be a new mom who thinks that a man is being selfish or making up an excuse to go out just to get away from you.

Be the smart new mom who trusts her husband, knows that he needs some space and relief from the anxieties of fatherhood, and is confident enough to know that giving a new dad permission to have "me" time is healthy for the marriage.

30
I need help networking with other dads

Although it is natural and socially acceptable for new moms to network with each other, new dads are uncomfortable and reluctant to connect with other dads to discuss their hopes, fears, and shortcomings with regard to fatherhood. As I noted in the Introduction, there are valid reasons for this. It all starts with the way our society raises boys. When a man becomes a new dad, the fear of being ridiculed by his male friends, coworkers, or employer still weighs heavily on his mind.

> "When I first heard that a class for dads was available, I wanted no part of it. Mainly because I didn't want my friends to know I was attending the class. But I'm glad I did."

"When the childbirth instructor announced the expectant dads class and invited the dads to attend, I could tell by the body language of the other guys that they were uncomfortable and had no interest. I went to make my wife happy."

"Attending a class for dads is just not something a guy advertises to other guys. Saying you're going to attend a group meeting gives the impression something is wrong in your life."

"I got enough flack from my friends for attending the childbirth classes and helping my wife around the house. If I tell them I'm attending a class for dads, I'll get more of the same."

"I work on the day the dads class is available. How do I justify taking a day off from work to attend a dads class? I'm afraid to ask my boss because I don't think he would approve of my reason for taking a day off or trading work days with a coworker."

"My father doesn't understand why I should pay for and attend a class for expectant dads. He thinks I'm a wimp and that the class is a waste of time. In his eyes, if he didn't attend a class, why should I?"

Another reason is the misconception new dads have about attending a fathering class with other dads.

"I have no desire to hang out with a bunch of guys for two hours who want to talk about their feelings."

"I'm not into any touchy-feely stuff and don't need anybody to give me a lecture on fatherhood."

"I'm already strapped for time with the childbirth classes. So I have no interest in a therapy session with a bunch of guys who want to talk about their feelings."

These dads' comments reflect the fear they have about people—especially male peers—questioning their masculinity or making them feel like less of a man.

The truth is that not all fathering programs are touchy-feely, therapy-based, or lecture-based sessions led by a professional counselor or therapist. Instead, the growing trend has been to establish informal forums led by your average dad. One such program is Boot Camp for New Dads (BCND) founded by Greg Bishop.

When Bishop pitched the idea to local hospitals, he was met with another unfortunate stigma about dads. The reactions to Bishop's proposal from hospital administrators and childbirth instructors were universal: "We don't believe dads will attend a class about fatherhood. It's not in their nature."

The response did not detour Bishop. He marched on and did not allow his detractors to keep him from his quest to provide this valuable, much-needed service for dads. He finally persuaded a local hospital in Irvine, California, to launch the program. Today there are over 250 BCND classes in forty-two states.

What makes BCND such a viable and unique program is that it incorporates veteran dads who return to class with their six-to-eight-week-old babies in the mix. If you are lucky enough to have a BCND program at your hospital, I highly recommend you encourage your husband to attend. After he graduates, he can pay it forward by returning to the class as a veteran dad with the baby and becoming a mentor for the new dads. Thanks to Bishop, another myth about dads has been dispelled.

There are many other informal programs like BCND for dads to choose from that provide a safe and interactive open-discussion forum for new dads. Check your local hospital and family resource centers or the Internet for more information.

Thanks to other fatherhood advocates and the Internet, since 1990 the dads network community has exploded. Other national fathering organizations include the National Fatherhood Initiative, National Center for Fathering, and Daddyshome, Inc. Several states have also established comprehensive fathering programs. And because of the Internet, informal support groups for dads have also grown exponentially. Two examples are the at-home-dad playgroups and dad blogs in operation nationwide. What the growth of these established dad groups proves is that dads are just as capable as moms when it comes to establishing a network system for themselves and other fathers.

Most new dads want to learn how to be better husbands and dads. Now that there is an established network available, all a new dad needs is words of encouragement and reassurance from his wife that connecting with other dads will benefit him. Share with him how much you've benefitted from your mom's network and how you view networking with other dads as a sign of courage.

Another way you can help your husband is to purchase the companion book *Pacifi(her): What She's Thinking When She's Pregnant.* This book will provide him with a dad's perspective and the courage to be more involved during the pregnancy.

If your husband is still reluctant to attend a class or join a network, encourage him to get together with one of the expectant dads in the childbirth class, or if you know an involved dad in the neighborhood, invite him to call your husband for a guy's night out. These dads can help break the ice and make your husband feel more comfortable about networking with other dads. If your husband is uncomfortable attending BCND or other expectant dads' classes by himself, he can invite, as other new dads have, his dad, father-in-law, friend, or a new dad he has met. With each new dad he meets, he will begin to realize that the best resource he has to become a better husband and dad is other dads. When he benefits, you and the baby will also reap the rewards, especially after the birth.